Physiology of Respiration

SECOND EDITION

Michael P. Hlastala, Ph.D.
*Professor of Physiology and Biophysics
and of
Medicine—Pulmonary and Critical Care*

Albert J. Berger, Ph.D.
Professor of Physiology and Biophysics

*School of Medicine
University of Washington
Seattle, Washington*

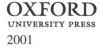

OXFORD
UNIVERSITY PRESS
2001

OXFORD
UNIVERSITY PRESS

Oxford   New York
Athens   Auckland   Bangkok   Bogotá   Buenos Aires   Calcutta
Cape Town   Chennai   Dar es Salaam   Delhi   Florence   Hong Kong   Istanbul
Karachi   Kuala Lumpur   Madrid   Melbourne   Mexico City   Mumbai   Nairobi
Paris   São Paulo   Shanghai   Singapore   Taipei   Tokyo   Toronto   Warsaw

and associated companies in
Berlin   Ibadan

Copyright © 2001 by Oxford University Press, Inc.

Published by Oxford University Press, Inc.
198 Madison Avenue, New York, New York 10016
http://www.oup-usa.org

Library of Congress Cataloging-in-Publication Data

Hlastala, Miachael P.
    Physiology of respiration / Michael P. Hlastala, Albert J. Berger.— 2nd ed.
    p. ; cm.
    Includes bibliographical references and index.
    ISBN 0-19-513846-5 (cloth : alk. paper) — ISBN 0-19-513847-3 (pbk. : alk. paper)
    1. Respiration.   2. Respiratory organs—Physiology.   I. Berger, Albert J.   II. Title.
    [DNLM: 1. Respiratory Physiology. WF 102 H677p 2001]
    QP121 .H68 2001
    612.2—dc21

                                                                              00-058039

1 3 5 7 9 8 6 4 2

Printed in the United States of America
on acid-free paper

To
Margaret, Marilyn
Dorian, Michael, Stefanie

Preface

Physiology of Respiration is written with the student in mind. Our intent in creating this work is to provide students with many of the modern ideas necessary to understand the broad subject of respiratory physiology. As such, it is an educational tool and not meant to be a compendium of the latest research findings. The scope of the book is comprehensive yet not overwhelming in the depth to which it covers any one topic. An important feature is that the two authors who wrote this book have diverse teaching and research interests in respiratory physiology. Thus, it provides not only up-to-date coverage of almost all major topics in respiratory physiology but also a unique, balanced perspective on these topics. Another important feature is the book's emphasis on underlying physiological mechanisms.

The second edition has undergone significant improvement based on input from readers of the first edition and new developments in the field. The order of the chapters has been changed to make the book more approachable by students. The development of some of the mathematical relationships has been moved to an appendix in Chapter 4 to simplify the learning process. The altitude and hyperbaric chapters have been combined into one (Chapter 11). Acid–base regulation (Chapter 13) has been simplified and is now located near the end of the book to reflect the respiratory system's key role in hydrogen ion regulation through CO_2 excretion by the lungs. This makes it important to understand respiratory physiology before learning about acid–base regulation. The comparative respiratory physiology chapter (Chapter 14) has been extensively revised to draw closer parallels to human respiratory physiology. Many old figures have been improved and new figures added. New concepts have been introduced into several chapters. These include new ideas about the distribution of lung blood flow and about respiratory rhythm generation.

Who should read this book? We feel it is appropriate for medical, dental, nursing, and other allied health students, as well as graduate students. This conclusion is based on a combined total of five decades of teaching this subject to all of these groups. In addition, scientists and clinicians who seek a text that will review basic information will find this to be a relevant source of such knowledge.

In so many ways, numerous people aided us in the creation of this work. We are particularly indebted to our teachers, mentors, and colleagues who taught us how to teach and write on this subject. Among these individuals are John Butler, Hazel Coleridge, John Coleridge, Julius H. Comroe, Leon Farhi, Ralph Kellogg, Claude Lenfant, Allen Mines, Robert A. Mitchell, Hermann Rahn, and Hugh Van Liew. We are particularly grateful to Jeffrey House of Oxford University Press for his long-term support in this endeavor.

Seattle, Wash.   M. P. H.

                                                                          A. J. B.

Contents

Physiology of Respiration

1

Overview and Physical Principles

Overview

The respiratory system is composed of the airways and lungs as well as the respiratory muscles that regulate gas movement into and out of these structures. Within the lungs, exchange of molecules of oxygen (O_2) and carbon dioxide (CO_2) between the gas and blood occurs.

The need for gas exchange is met in different ways by various organisms. In single-cell organisms, it can be met by simple molecular diffusion across the cell membrane to and from the external environment. There is no need for specialized gas exchange or a blood-pumping and distribution system. It has been estimated that this strategy may be adequate for spherical-shaped organisms no larger than 1 mm in diameter.

Larger, multicellular organisms require circulatory and respiratory gas exchange systems. Such systems are found throughout the animal kingdom. For example, insects have developed infoldings of their body walls that form networks of tube-like airways called *tracheae*. These tracheae bring external air into close proximity with the cells that require exchange of O_2 and CO_2. In fish, the respiratory gas exchange system comprises gills, which are turned outward into the water environment. Gills are delicate and dry out quickly when exposed to air. Movement of water across the gills facilitates the exchange of O_2 and CO_2. Another example of a specialized exchange system is the lungs. Here the respiratory exchange apparatus is turned inward, creating an infolded cavity. External air is warmed and also humidified before it arrives at the gas-exchanging regions of the lungs. Thus there is a whole host of strategies for solving the problem of efficient gas exchange with the environment.

The primary function of the respiratory system is to deliver sufficient amounts of O_2 from the external environment to the tissues. Thus blood emerging from the lungs on its way to the tissues must be adequately and efficiently oxygenated (Fig. 1.1). "Adequately" means that the level of O_2 in the arterial blood must be sufficient to meet the body's metabolic demands; "efficiently" means that the energy costs of breathing (work done by the respiratory muscles in moving gas in and out of the lungs) and of pumping blood through the pulmonary circulation are kept as low as possible. After leaving the pulmonary circulation, the oxygenated blood is delivered via the left heart to the tissue capillary beds, where O_2 is first unloaded from the blood and then is passed by diffusion to cells requiring this energy substrate.

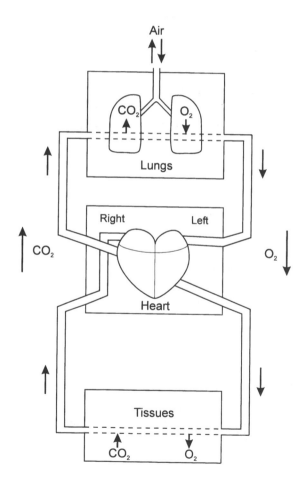

Figure 1.1. Schematic diagram showing the flow of O_2 from the environment through the lungs to tissues and the flow of CO_2 from tissues through the lungs to the environment.

Another major gas exchange function of the respiratory system is to remove CO_2 that is produced by cellular metabolism. In some ways, this process is the reverse of the O_2 delivery problem. Carbon dioxide moves by diffusion from cells to the capillaries, where it is then transported by blood via the right heart to the lungs for release into the atmosphere in the exhaled gas.

There is an important issue to consider when thinking about a highly integrated system such as the human respiratory system: What are the variables that are regulated so that the system can function optimally? In the respiratory system, ventilation is regulated by rhythmic contractions of the respiratory muscles; these contractions arise from neural signals emerging from the central nervous system. Pulmonary blood flow is also a regulated variable and is set primarily by the pumping action of the heart. Clearly, coordination of the cardiovascular and respiratory systems is necessary for the efficient exchange of the respiratory gases, O_2 and CO_2. During exercise, for example, when the demand for O_2 and the production of CO_2 are elevated, increasing the blood flow is simply not sufficient to meet these demands without also increasing pulmonary ventilation. If blood flow is increased during exercise without increased ventilation, the result will be a reduction in the partial pressure of O_2 and an elevation in the partial pressure of CO_2 in blood emerging from the lungs. This clearly would result in the arterial blood delivering insufficient O_2 to exercising muscles. Thus an appropriate strategy that occurs normally is for cardiac output and pulmonary ventilation *each* to increase proportionally to meet the demands of increased O_2 consumption and CO_2 production.

The human respiratory system is subject to diseases that can markedly alter its gas-exchanging function. An understanding of the pathophysiology helps make clear that it is the matching of ventilation to perfusion within the gas-exchanging regions of the lungs that is paramount in determining the efficiency of the gas exchange process. Poorly ventilated, highly perfused lung regions, together with regions that are highly ventilated but poorly perfused, result in less efficient blood gas exchange. A hallmark of chronic obstructive pulmonary diseases, such as asthma, chronic bronchitis, and emphysema, is airflow obstruction. If gas flow in the airways is reduced due to inflammation, mucus-plugging, narrowing, or loss of elastic recoil of the airways, then ventilation will be reduced. As a consequence, matching of ventilation to blood flow in the lungs will be altered so that gas exchange is compromised, and this will cause the arterial O_2 partial pressure to fall (hypoxemia) and the CO_2 partial pressure to rise (hypercapnia). Under such circumstances, clinical strategies are called for to improve the matching of ventilation to blood flow in the lungs. An understanding of the basic physical principles that govern the physiology of the respiratory system will provide a basis for learning how these strategies work.

Physical Principles—Gases

Knowledge of the physical laws that govern the behavior of gases and liquids is critical to the understanding of respiratory physiology. The basic principles used in this book are introduced here in the hope that encountering them at the beginning of your study of respiratory physiology will facilitate their mastery.

Movement of gases into and out of the lungs is essential for respiration. A gas consists of molecules that have considerable random mobility and no fixed spatial relationships between molecules. A gas will completely fill a container or volume in which it is confined. This characteristic contrasts with that of a liquid or a solid, which, because of greater intermolecular forces, will not fully occupy a container, unless of course the volume of the liquid or the solid is equal to the volume of its container.

Pressure

An important concept when considering the behavior of gases is pressure. The pressure of a gas is directly proportional to the average force per unit area that the gas molecules exert on the wall of their container. Pressure is generated by collision of gas molecules with the container wall.

The total pressure exerted by the gas molecules of the atmosphere is termed the *barometric pressure* (P_B). The basic pressure unit used in respiratory physiology is the millimeter of mercury (abbreviated mm Hg). An alternative pressure unit, employed in the modern metric system of units (so-called SI units), is the kilopascal (kPa).* At sea level, P_B is 760 mm Hg† or 101 kPa. Because the density of the atmosphere is lower at higher altitudes, P_B declines with increasing altitude (see Chapter 11). To make calculations involving small changes in gas pressures, such as pressure differences responsible for the flow of gas into and out of the lungs, pressure is expressed relative to atmospheric pressure; this relative pressure is termed "gauge pressure." For example, an absolute pressure of 755 mm Hg in the alveoli when the ambient atmospheric pressure is 760 mm Hg would be expressed as −5 mm Hg. Furthermore, for those measurements involving small pressure differences, another pressure unit is used, the centimeter of water (cm H_2O), which has greater sensitivity than the mm Hg unit. It is convenient to remember that there

---

*Because pressure is a force per unit area and force is mass times acceleration, the SI unit of pressure is the newton · m^{-2}, and this is called the *pascal*. The *kilopascal* is 1000 pascals (kPa), and 1 kPa is equivalent to 7.50 mm Hg.

†Standard atmospheric pressure raises a column of mercury in an evacuated tube to a height of 760 mm (29.92 inches).

is 1.36 cm H_2O for every 1 mm Hg of pressure. This is derived from the ratio between the densities of mercury (13.6 gm $\cdot$ cm^{-3}) and water (1 gm $\cdot$ cm^{-3}).

Pressure is directly proportional to the kinetic energy of gas molecules. As such, the higher the temperature, the greater will be the kinetic energy and therefore also the pressure of the gas within a container of fixed volume in which it is confined. Another important concept regarding gas pressure is that the greater the number of gas molecules in a given volume, the higher the pressure. This is because the more gas molecules that are present, the greater the average number of collisions occurring with the wall of the container per unit time. Finally, if the volume of the container is reduced without changing either the temperature or the number of molecules of gas, the average number of collisions per unit time will increase, and so will the pressure.

Ideal Gas Law

The intuitive concepts concerning the behavior of gases with relation to changing conditions are the basis for the ideal gas law. This gas law is really two separate laws—*Boyle's law* and *Charles' law*. Boyle's law states that for a constant absolute temperature and number of gas molecules, the pressure and volume are reciprocally related one to the other. Thus, the doubling of a volume of a gas will halve its pressure. Charles' law states that at a constant pressure and number of gas molecules, the volume occupied by a gas is directly proportional to the absolute temperature. Thus a doubling of the absolute temperature will double the volume occupied by a gas. The ideal gas law expresses the relationship between pressure (P, units of atmospheres or mm Hg); volume (V, units of liters [l]); absolute temperature (T, units of degrees Kelvin, which is 273°K plus the temperature in degrees or Celsius); the number of moles of gas (n); and the gas constant, which is a proportionality constant (R, units of 0.08205 l $\cdot$ atmosphere $\cdot$ mole^{-1} $\cdot$ degree^{-1}, or 62.32 l $\cdot$ mm Hg $\cdot$ mole^{-1} $\cdot$ degree^{-1})

$$PV = nRT \qquad (1.1)$$

The ideal gas law applies when the total pressure is low. This means specifically that the individual gas molecules can be treated as isolated points in space, having negligible molecular volume and exerting no intermolecular forces other than those resulting from perfectly elastic collisions between molecules. This is a reasonable assumption at the low pressures normally encountered in respiratory physiology because, under these conditions, the average intermolecular distance is about ten times the average molecular size. The ideal gas law, therefore, reasonably describes the behavior of respiratory gases. At very high pressures the behavior of gases deviates from the ideal gas law because the intermolecular distances become reduced.

From the ideal gas law one can determine the volume occupied by a mole of gas at 0°C and 1 atmosphere of pressure (760 mm Hg). Under these conditions, the volume is 22.4 l. Thus, any mole of an ideal gas—independent of the type—will occupy the same volume, given these conditions of temperature and pressure. For example, 1 gm-mole of N_2 (molecular weight [MW] = 28.0 gm · gm-mole^{-1}) or O_2 (MW = 32.0 gm · gm-mole^{-1}) each will occupy 22.4 l at 0°C and 760 mm Hg. Another handy physical constant that is important when using the ideal gas law is the number of molecules that are present in a gram-mole. This is called *Avogadro's number* and is 6.023×10^{23}.

Thus 22.4 l of any ideal gas at the standard conditions of 0°C and 1 atmosphere pressure will contain 6.023×10^{23} molecules.

Dalton's Law of Partial Pressures

The air we breathe is a mixture of several molecular species. Table 1.1 lists the primary components and their concentrations assuming that the air is dry. For practical purposes, it is usual to assume that air contains 21% O_2 and 79% N_2, with other inert gases, such as argon, being lumped into the N_2 portion. The CO_2 component in the air is also ignored because its concentration is relatively small. In a gas mixture, the pressure exerted by each individual gas species is referred to as its *partial pressure* (P). If a gas mixture is enclosed in a sealed container (Fig. 1.2), it will develop a pressure by means of molecular collisions of the gas with the container wall. The partial pressure of any component of gas is the pressure developed by the molecules of that component acting alone, that is, as if it were occupying the entire volume of the container by itself. This view of the gas mixture

Table 1.1. Primary Components of Dry Air

SPECIES	CONTENT IN VOLUME PERCENT
Nitrogen	78.08
Oxygen	20.95
Carbon dioxide	0.03
Argon	0.93

Data do not include water vapor. Also not shown are trace components, including neon, helium, krypton, xenon, hydrogen, methane, and nitrous oxide. (Data from DR Lide, editor. CRC—*Handbook of Chemistry and Physics*, 71st ed. Boca Raton, FL: CRC Press, 1990.)

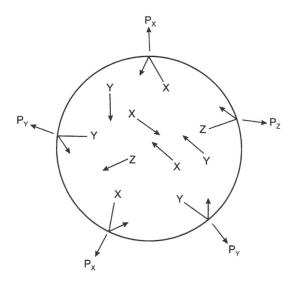

Figure 1.2. A sphere containing 10 molecules of gases of three different species, X, Y, Z. Each gas exerts a pressure (P) on the surface of the sphere that is proportional to the number of molecules of that gas contained within the sphere.

assumes that the gas molecules act independently, which they do at low gas pressures.

This principle of independent action of each gas is the basis for Dalton's law of partial pressures, which states that the total pressure of a gas mixture (P_t) is equal to the sum of the partial pressures of all the gases in the mixture. The following relationship applies to the gases present within the lungs:

$$P_t = P_{CO_2} + P_{O_2} + P_{N_2} + P_{H_2O} \tag{1.2}$$

(Note that the P_{CO_2} is not ignored because it is much higher in the lungs than in air.)

Another important relationship is that the partial pressure of a gas (P_X) can be expressed in terms of the fractional concentration (F_X) of that gas multiplied by the total pressure:

$$P_X = F_X \times P_t \tag{1.3}$$

where X represents a single gas species. For example, this relationship can be used to determine the partial pressure of O_2 in the air. Because the fraction of O_2 in air is 0.21, its partial pressure will be

$$P_{O_2} = 0.21 \times 760 \text{ mm Hg} = 160 \text{ mm Hg}$$

Vapor Pressure

When a liquid is exposed to open space above its surface, molecules of dissolved gas will escape from the liquid surface into the space above. Equilibrium is reached when the rate of escape of molecules from the liquid phase equals the rate at which gas molecules reenter the liquid phase. The vapor pressure of a gas over a liquid is the partial pressure exerted by gas molecules when there is an equilibrium between the liquid and gas phases for these molecules. In respiratory physiology, the most common vapor pressure measured is that for water. At equilibrium, the partial pressure of water in the gas phase is equal to its vapor pressure. The vapor pressure of water is solely dependent on temperature. For example, at a body temperature of 37°C the vapor pressure of water is 47 mm Hg, whereas at the boiling point of water (100°C) it is 760 mm Hg. Thus the higher the temperature, the greater the vapor pressure of water, because the kinetic energy of the liquid water molecules increases and, as a consequence, the rate at which molecules escape from the surface also increases. Figure 1.3 shows the vapor pressure of water between 0° and 50°C, which covers much of the range encountered in physiological studies.

A commonly used quantitative measure of the amount of water in air is the *relative humidity*, which is defined as the ratio of the measured partial pressure of water in the air to the vapor pressure of water, which is determined solely by the temperature of the air (Fig. 1.3). For example, if the relative humidity is 50% at a

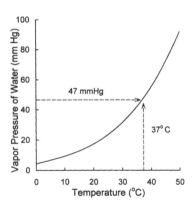

Temperature °C	Vapor Pressure mmHg	Vapor Pressure kPa
0	4.6	0.61
10	9.2	1.23
20	17.5	2.33
30	31.8	4.24
37	47.0	6.27
40	55.3	7.37
50	92.5	12.33

Figure 1.3. Relationship between the vapor pressure of water and temperature. Arrows indicate the vapor pressure at normal body temperature. Also shown is a table with selected values of vapor pressure of water as a function of temperature.

temperature of 20°C (at this temperature the vapor pressure of water is 17.5 mm Hg [see Fig. 1.3]), then the partial pressure of water will be

$$P_{H_2O} = (0.5) \times 17.5 \text{ mm Hg} = 8.75 \text{ mm Hg}$$

Although the air we breathe is almost always cooler than normal body temperature, its water content rarely is 100% saturated (i.e., 100% relative humidity). Inspired air entering the respiratory system is warmed to body temperature and humidified to full saturation by exchange of heat and water from the airway surfaces. Under these conditions (and using Dalton's law), if P_B is 760 mm Hg and P_{H_2O} is 47 mm Hg, the difference of 713 mm Hg is the sum of the partial pressures of all the remaining inspired gases. Of this total, 21% is O_2 and 79% is N_2. After the inspired gas is warmed and humidified, inspired P_{O_2} (PI_{O_2}) can be calculated as follows:

$$\begin{aligned} PI_{O_2} &= FI_{O_2}(P_B - P_{H_2O}) \\ &= 0.21 \times (760 - 47) = 0.21 \times 713 \\ &= 150 \text{ mm Hg} \end{aligned} \tag{1.4}$$

Therefore, due to the warming of the inspired air and its saturation with water vapor in moving from outside ambient conditions, where it is dry, to within the airways, the P_{O_2} drops by approximately 10 mm Hg. Thus, the inspired air that enters the alveoli with each breath has a P_{O_2} that is reduced by this amount compared with the inspired air that enters the nose and mouth.

Conversion Between Conditions

In respiratory physiology, gas volumes are measured under different conditions of temperature, pressure, and degrees of saturation with water vapor. The three most common conditions are (*1*) ambient temperature and pressure, saturated (ATPS); (*2*) body temperature, ambient pressure, saturated (BTPS); and (*3*) standard temperature and pressure, dry (STPD). To give some examples, the ATPS conditions are encountered when exhaled gas is collected in a spirometer or bag; BTPS conditions constitute ventilatory volumes actually measured within the lungs; and the STPD condition is used to express rates of consumption or production of respiratory gases ($\dot{V}$), such as the metabolic consumption rate of O_2 ($\dot{V}_{O_2}$) and metabolic production rate of CO_2 ($\dot{V}_{CO_2}$), which customarily are measured at a pressure of 760 mm Hg and 0°C. Conversions between the various conditions (e.g., between state 1 and state 2 where the same number of moles of gas exists in each state) can be made by using the following relationship based on the ideal gas law:

$$\frac{V_1(P_1 - P_{1H_2O})}{T_1} = \frac{V_2(P_2 - P_{2H_2O})}{T_2} \qquad (1.5)$$

Conversions to dry conditions can be made by setting the partial pressure of water vapor to zero. It follows from these relations that when changing from ATPS to BTPS there is a volume expansion of approximately 10% over the ambient condition.

Gas Solubility

The solubility of gases in liquids is important to our understanding of blood gas transport mechanisms. The amount of gas that can dissolve in a liquid is directly proportional to the partial pressure of that gas above the liquid. This is a statement of an important physical law termed *Henry's law*. It is important to distinguish the amount of gas dissolved in the liquid from that which may *chemically* combine with the liquid. Henry's law refers only to the quantity of gas that is *dissolved* at equilibrium, when the partial pressures of a given species in the gas and liquid phases are equal. Henry's law is described by the following relationship:

$$C_X = \beta_X \, P_X \qquad (1.6)$$

Here again, X denotes a single gas species, and C_X represents the concentration of dissolved species now in the liquid phase. Typical units for this quantity (of gases dissolved in blood) are milliliters (ml) of dissolved gas at STPD per deciliter (dl; 100 ml) of blood (also termed *volume percent*). The proportional factor, $(\beta_X$, is the solubility coefficient. Its units are milliliters of dissolved gas at STPD per deciliter of blood per mm Hg. The solubility coefficient depends on temperature; the higher the temperature, the smaller its value. Thus, at a higher temperature, less gas will dissolve in a given volume of liquid.

The following example illustrates the use of Henry's law to calculate the concentration of dissolved O_2 in plasma when the surface of the plasma is exposed to fully saturated air. At 20°C, the O_2 solubility coefficient is 0.00364 ml $O_2 \cdot dl^{-1} \cdot$ mm Hg^{-1}, and, as calculated above, the P_{O_2} is 150 mm Hg; therefore,

$$C_{O_2} = 0.00364 \text{ ml } O_2 \cdot dl^{-1} \cdot \text{mm } Hg^{-1} \times 150 \text{ mm Hg}$$
$$= 0.55 \text{ ml } O_2 \cdot dl^{-1}$$

If the temperature is raised to a body temperature of 37°C, the solubility coefficient drops to 0.00282 ml $O_2 \cdot dl^{-1} \cdot$ mm Hg^{-1}, and the amount of dissolved O_2 is now 0.42 ml $O_2 \cdot dl^{-1}$. This example illustrates how little O_2 is actually dissolved in plasma under normal body conditions and why the O_2 transporting molecule hemoglobin is needed for blood to carry sufficient O_2 to the tissues. Also, the amount of O_2 dissolved is sensitive to temperature, decreasing by 22% when going from a room temperature of 20°C to a body temperature of 37°C.

Physical Principles—Flow of Fluids

The flow of fluids, whether they be gas or liquid, occurs because of pressure differences—that is, a fluid will flow from a higher pressure to a lower pressure. Analogously, by using *Ohm's law* for the flow of electricity (difference in electrical potential = current × electrical resistance), the following relationships among fluid flow ($\dot{V}$), pressure difference ($\Delta P = P_1 - P_2$), and flow resistance (R) apply (see also Fig. 1.4A):

A. Overall Flow

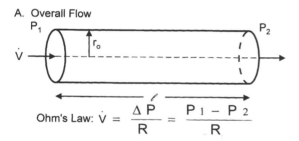

Ohm's Law: $\dot{V} = \dfrac{\Delta P}{R} = \dfrac{P_1 - P_2}{R}$

B. Laminar Flow

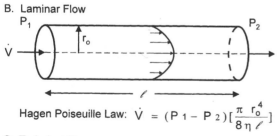

Hagen Poiseuille Law: $\dot{V} = (P_1 - P_2)[\dfrac{\pi\, r_0^4}{8\eta\, \ell}]$

C. Turbulent Flow

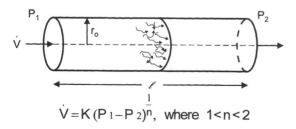

$\dot{V} = K(P_1 - P_2)^{\frac{1}{n}}$, where $1 < n < 2$

Figure 1.4. A, Ohm's law analogy for flow of a fluid in a tube. **B,** Velocity profile for laminar flow and Hagen-Poiseuille law. **C,** Turbulent flow and the empirical relationship for the overall flow. See text for a discussion of the variables indicated. In **B** and **C** the time average velocity profile is indicated by the curved line in the middle of the flow tube; streamlines also are indicated by small arrows.

$$\text{Force} = \text{Flow} \times \text{Resistance} \qquad (1.7)$$

$$\Delta P = \dot{V} \times R \qquad (1.8)$$

Rearranging equation 1.8 yields

$$\dot{V} = \frac{\Delta P}{R} \qquad (1.9)$$

Thus, at a constant R, if the pressure difference is doubled, for example, by increasing the upstream pressure [P_1], then $\dot{V}$ will double. This relationship also illustrates that if flow resistance is halved (e.g., by increasing the radius of a tube through which the fluid is flowing), the result is a doubling of flow for a constant ΔP. In respiratory physiology, R has important implications because it indicates, for example, the degree of constriction of the airways. Airway narrowing that is due to a disease process, such as asthma, can be assessed by measuring airway resistance.

The Ohm's law analogy for fluid flow that is described above readily lends itself to a consideration of series and parallel flow resistances. In the respiratory system, air flow resistance of the nasal airways is in series with the resistance across the larynx. Thus, when considered together, the total resistance is simply the sum of the two individual resistances. In general, total flow resistance (R_t) is the sum of the individual flow resistances in series and can be described as follows:

$$R_t = R_1 + R_2 + \ldots + R_i + \ldots + R_N = \sum_{i=1}^{N} R_i \qquad (1.10)$$

Flow resistances also occur in parallel. For example, pulmonary blood flow to the right and left lungs is a parallel system. In this situation, the overall pulmonary blood flow resistance is equal to one divided by the sum of the reciprocal of each of the resistances. In general terms, flow resistances in parallel are defined by the following equation:

$$R_t = \frac{1}{\displaystyle\sum_{i=1}^{N} \frac{1}{R_i}} \qquad (1.11)$$

From equation 1.11 it is apparent that the addition of a parallel flow resistance will reduce the total resistance. In contrast, when a series resistance is added, the overall resistance increases.

Flow that occurs when a fluid goes through a rigid tube generally is one of two types, laminar flow or turbulent flow. There are a number of differences between them. First, laminar flow involves less dissipation of energy than does turbulent flow, and consequently for a given flow rate, less energy (i.e., a lower pressure drop) is required to move the fluid. In steady laminar flow, each particle of fluid flows linearly, parallel to the overall direction of flow. Streamlines indicate the paths taken by the flowing fluid particles. In Figure 1.4B, the streamlines of fluid flow can be seen parallel to the direction of flow. In turbulent flow, a very different picture of flow emerges in which there is a mixing of fluid over the cross-sectional area of the conduit (Fig. 1.4C). Thus, whereas the direction of time-averaged flow is from high pressure to low, the instantaneous flow velocity and streamlines at any one point may be aimed in *any* direction. Turbulent flow is characteristic of higher flow velocities; it is more likely to occur where there is a rough inner surface or a bend in the conduit.

For laminar flow, the overall flow rate can be explicitly determined (Fig. 1.4B). In a rigid tube with a circular cross section, the flow velocity profile, when fully developed, is described by a parabola, and maximal velocity occurs at the center of the tube. For time-invariant flow of a noncompressible fluid in a rigid tube of circular cross section, the overall flow rate is expressed as follows by the *Hagen-Poiseuille law*:

$$\dot{V} = (P_1 - P_2) \left[\frac{\pi r_o^4}{8\eta\ell} \right] \tag{1.12}$$

where r_o is the radius of the tube, η is the viscosity, and ℓ is the length of the tube. Thus $\dot{V}$ is strongly dependent on r_o. For example, halving of the radius results in a drop in flow rate to 1/16 of its original value if all other variables are constant. From equations 1.9 and 1.12, we can deduce that the resistance to flow (R) is proportional to η and ℓ and inversely proportional to r_o^4. In the small peripheral airways the airflow is laminar, and therefore the Hagen-Poiseuille law adequately predicts the relationships among the variables just described, $\dot{V}$ and the pressure drop.

As $\dot{V}$ increases, flow becomes turbulent. Turbulent flow occurs in the larger central airways, including the bronchi, as well as in the upper airways, including the nose, pharynx, larynx, and trachea. The point of transition between laminar and turbulent flow is predicted by a dimensionless number called the *Reynolds number* (N_{Re}). The Reynolds number is

$$N_{Re} = \frac{2r_o v\rho}{\eta} \tag{1.13}$$

where v is the average flow velocity and ρ is the density. The transition between laminar and turbulent flow occurs at an N_{Re} of about 2100, assuming that the flow is incompressible, is at steady state, and is occurring within a straight smooth tube. If bends are present, if the tube bifurcates, or if the tube's surface is rough, such as occurs in the large airways, then the transition between fully developed laminar and turbulent flows does not occur at a specific N_{Re}. This transitional flow zone is described as being between fully developed laminar and turbulent flow regimes.

The prediction of the relationship between $\dot{V}$ and ΔP for turbulent flow is empirical. A good approximation is presented in Figure 1.4C. In the turbulent zone, the flow is proportional to the pressure drop raised to a power of less than 1. Now a doubling of the flow, when flow is turbulent, will require more than a doubling of the pressure drop. Recall that in laminar flow (Eq. 1.12) a doubling of flow involves a doubling of pressure drop. Furthermore, compared with laminar flow, the turbulent flow velocity profile—which is the time-averaged velocity measured at any point—is much flatter; but, as in laminar flow, the time-averaged maximal velocity also occurs at the center of the tube.

Physical Principles—Mass Balances

The *conservation of mass principle* is of paramount importance in understanding the respiratory system. It is used, for example, in determining consumption and production of O_2 and CO_2, respectively, and in determining blood flow rates. In general, for any species within a system, the mass balance relationship is the following:

Rate of accumulation of the species within the system	=	Total rate of inflow of the species to the system	−	Total rate of outflow of the species from the system	+	Rate of production of the species within the system

An easy way to understand the conservation of mass is to apply it to some examples, keeping in mind that the units of each of the terms could be in mass · time^{-1}, moles · time^{-1}, or (ml of gas) · time^{-1}. While all these units are acceptable, it is critical when using the above relationship that each of the terms has the same units.

As an example, first consider the flow of a species, X, across the wall of a capillary. In this case the system is defined by a boundary (dashed line in Fig. 1.5) enclosing the inflow, outflow, and diffusive flow of the species across the wall of the capillary. In this simple example there is no production of the species within the system boundary. Furthermore, we will consider the system to be in a steady

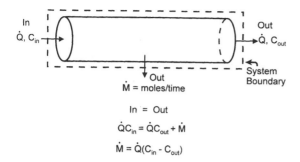

$$In = Out$$

$$\dot{Q}C_{in} = \dot{Q}C_{out} + \dot{M}$$

$$\dot{M} = \dot{Q}(C_{in} - C_{out})$$

Figure 1.5. Diagram illustrating mass balance across a capillary. See text for a discussion of the variables indicated.

state so that there is a time-invariant balance of what is flowing into and what is flowing out of the system for the species X. This simplification means that the rate of accumulation of X within the system is zero. Therefore, the above expression reduces to the following:

$$0 = \begin{matrix} \text{Total rate} \\ \text{of inflow} \\ \text{of the species} \\ \text{to the system} \end{matrix} - \begin{matrix} \text{Total rate of} \\ \text{outflow of the} \\ \text{species from} \\ \text{the system} \end{matrix} + 0$$

Or:

$$\begin{matrix} \text{Total rate} \\ \text{of inflow} \\ \text{of the species} \\ \text{to the system} \end{matrix} = \begin{matrix} \text{Total rate of} \\ \text{outflow of the} \\ \text{species from} \\ \text{the system} \end{matrix}$$

From Figure 1.5 the mass balance indicates that the mass flow rate of species X, which leaves by diffusion ($\dot{M}$) through the capillary wall, is equal to the blood flow rate ($\dot{Q}$) times the concentration difference across the capillary:

$$\dot{M} = \dot{Q} (C_{in} - C_{out}) \qquad (1.14)$$

The above expression is a very important one and is termed *Fick's principle*. For example, this principle can be used to calculate the total cardiac blood flow if one knows the rate at which O_2 is taken up from the blood perfusing the tissues of the body ($\dot{V}_{O_2}$) and the arterial (a) − venous (v) oxygen concentration difference. In this instance, equation 1.14 is solved for $\dot{Q}$, the total cardiac output, thus yielding other forms of Fick's principle:

$$\dot{Q} = \frac{\dot{M}}{C_{in} - C_{out}} \tag{1.15}$$

Or

$$\dot{Q} = \frac{\dot{V}_{O_2}}{Ca_{O_2} - Cv_{O_2}} \tag{1.16}$$

By measuring the overall O_2 consumption per unit time (250 ml $O_2 \cdot min^{-1}$) and the arterial (200 ml $O_2 \cdot 1$ blood^{-1}) and venous (150 ml $O_2 \cdot 1$ blood^{-1}) O_2 concentrations (Ca_{O_2} and Cv_{O_2}, respectively), one can calculate the overall cardiac output:

$$\dot{Q} = \frac{250 \text{ ml } O_2 \cdot min^{-1}}{200 \text{ ml } O_2 \cdot 1^{-1} - 150 \text{ ml } O_2 \cdot 1^{-1}} \tag{1.17}$$

$$\dot{Q} = \frac{250}{50} 1 \cdot min^{-1} = 5 \ 1 \cdot min^{-1} \tag{1.18}$$

Another variation of the conservation of mass principle can be used to determine an unknown volume. To do this, a known amount of a dye or indicator is introduced into the unknown volume. The unknown volume can now be calculated by determining the concentration of dye or indicator within the volume after it has become uniformly distributed. As described in Chapter 3, the lungs contain a volume of gas that cannot be exhaled no matter how hard one tries; this volume is termed the *residual volume*. A common clinical method to determine this volume is to introduce a known amount of a poorly blood-soluble trace component, such as the inert gas helium, into the inhaled gas and after equilibration of this component with the gas in the lungs, to measure the concentration of helium in the lungs; from this information the residual volume is calculated with the conservation of mass principle.

In summary, the conservation of mass principle is applied in many situations that commonly occur in clinical respiratory physiology. The important points to keep in mind when applying this principle are (*1*) the boundary that defines the system over which the conservation of mass is applied must be carefully specified; (*2*) the units of each term in the conservation of mass relationship must express the same units such as moles $\cdot$ time^{-1}; (*3*) finally, all terms in the general expression must be utilized, when appropriate, to account for conservation of the species of interest.

Physical Principles—Diffusion

Molecular diffusion within gases and liquids is an important biological process that accounts for most mass transport that occurs at the cellular level. Small, simple organisms use diffusion almost exclusively to obtain the necessary metabolic substrates and to remove the waste products of metabolism. Complex organisms, such as humans, use molecular diffusion in conjunction with forced convection, as in the respiratory and cardiovascular systems.

By the term *molecular diffusion* we mean the transport of a species from a region of high concentration or partial pressure to one of low concentration or partial pressure within a single phase such as a liquid or a gas. The equation that describes the rate of molecular diffusion through a barrier, such as a membrane, is *Fick's first law of diffusion*. Figure 1.6 illustrates this relationship and shows that the mass flow rate per unit time ($\dot{M}_x$) is directly proportional to the cross-sectional area (A) across which diffusion occurs, inversely proportional to the thickness of the membrane (ℓ) and directly proportional to the concentration driving force across the membrane. The proportionality factor is the diffusion coefficient ($\mathcal{D}$), which indicates the mobility of the species within the membrane. The units of $\mathcal{D}$ are $cm^2 \cdot sec^{-1}$.

Several important concepts emerge when considering Fick's law of diffusion. First, this is a linear model; thus $\dot{M}_x$ is linearly related to the concentration driving

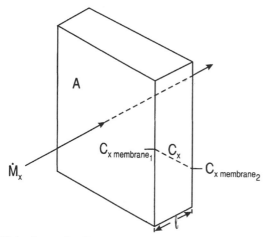

Fick's Law of Diffusion:

$$\dot{M}_x = \frac{-\mathcal{D}A}{\ell}(C_{x\,membrane_1} - C_{x\,membrane_2})$$

Figure 1.6. Diagram illustrating mass transport across membrane. Concentration (C_x) of transported species (X) is the same for the well-stirred bulk fluid as it is on the membrane surface. Also indicated is Fick's law of diffusion relating mass flow rate ($\dot{M}_x$) to diffusivity ($\mathcal{D}$), cross-sectional area of the membrane (A), membrane thickness (ℓ), and concentration difference across the membrane ($C_{X\,membrane_1} - C_{X\,membrane_2}$).

force, and it is not dependent on either the absolute value of C_X or the presence of other species in the system.

Second, $\mathcal{D}$ is related to a number of physical quantities. In one model of diffusion, called the *hydrodynamical theory* (which is based on diffusion of large spherical molecules in a liquid medium), $\mathcal{D}$ is directly proportional to the absolute temperature and inversely proportional to the radius of the diffusing molecule. Thus, as temperature increases, diffusion will increase, and as the size of the diffusing molecule increases, diffusion will decrease. Concerning this latter relationship, the size of a molecule is related to its molecular weight. Therefore, as an approximation, molecules of higher molecular weight will diffuse more slowly than molecules of lower molecular weight. This concept arises from *Graham's law*, which states that the rate of diffusion of a gas is inversely related to its density.

Third, Fick's law of diffusion (described in Fig. 1.6) considers the concentration of the diffusing species only in the surface of the membrane and not in the bulk fluid overlying the surface. A substance will have a solubility just within the surface of the membrane, which is dependent on, but not equal to, its concentration in the fluid overlying the membrane surface. Therefore, although we can measure the concentration of the substance in the overlying fluid, we cannot easily deduce the concentration in the membrane. To circumvent this problem and arrive at a relationship similar to that given in Figure 1.6 for Fick's law of diffusion, we can utilize the partition coefficient (λ_X), which relates the concentrations in the membrane surface to that in the overlying fluid:

$$\lambda_X = \frac{C_{X\ \text{membrane}}}{C_{X\ \text{fluid}}} \tag{1.19}$$

If we solve equation 1.19 for the concentration in the membrane surface and put this into Fick's law of diffusion (shown in Fig. 1.6), assuming that λ_X is the same on both sides of the membrane, the following relationship results:

$$\dot{M}_X = \frac{-\mathcal{D}A\lambda_X}{\ell} \left(C_{X\ \text{fluid}_1} - C_{X\ \text{fluid}_2} \right) \tag{1.20}$$

The concentrations are now those in the overlying medium. Equation 1.20 can be further simplified by defining the permeability ($\mathcal{P}_X$) of a species as the following:

$$\mathcal{P}_X = \frac{\mathcal{D}\lambda_X}{\ell} \tag{1.21}$$

This results in the following expression:

$$\dot{M}_X = -\mathcal{P}_X A \left(C_{X\ \text{fluid}_1} - C_{X\ \text{fluid}_2} \right) \tag{1.22}$$

Thus, even when the concentration of a species within the surface of a membrane is not equal to that in the fluid overlying the membrane, the overall diffusion rate will be simply related to the concentration differences in the medium on both sides of the membrane.

Further Reading

1. Bird RB, Stewart WE, Lightfoot EN. *Transport Phenomena*. New York: John Wiley & Sons, 1960.
2. Cameron JN. *The Respiratory Physiology of Animals*. New York: Oxford University Press, 1989, pp 2–35.
3. Chang HK. Diffusion of gases. In: Farhi LE, Tenney SM, editors. *Handbook of Physiology*. Section 3, *The Respiratory System*, vol. IV, *Gas Exchange*. Bethesda, MD: American Physiological Society, 1987, pp 33–50.
4. Kellogg RH. Laws of physics pertaining to gas exchange. In: Farhi LE, Tenney SM, editors. *Handbook of Physiology*. Section 3, *The Respiratory System*, vol IV, *Gas Exchange*. Bethesda, MD: American Physiological Society, 1987, pp 13–31.
5. LaBarbera M. Principles of design of fluid transport systems in zoology. *Science* 249: 992–1000, 1990.

Study Questions

1.1. What is the partial pressure of a gas?

1.2. What is the equilibrium vapor pressure of a gas over a liquid?

1.3. The amount of gas that can dissolve in a liquid is directly proportional to what variable?

1.4. How much O_2 will dissolve in plasma if the solubility coefficient of O_2 in plasma at 37°C is 0.00282 ml $O_2 \cdot dl^{-1} \cdot$ mm Hg^{-1} and the O_2 partial pressure is 100mm Hg?

1.5. In a flow system, what will the addition of a parallel flow resistance do to the total resistance? What will the addition of a series flow resistance do to the total resistance?

1.6. In laminar flow in a tube, the resistance to flow is inversely proportional to what power of the radius? How will the resistance change if the radius is halved?

1.7. If a subject's overall O_2 consumption per unit time is 200 ml $O_2 \cdot min^{-1}$, his cardiac output is 5(l) $\cdot min^{-1}$, and the venous O_2 concentration is 150 ml $O_2 \cdot$ (l) $blood^{-1}$, what will be his arterial O_2 concentration?

1.8. What is meant by *molecular diffusion*?

1.9. Based on Fick's law of diffusion, how is the mass flow rate per unit time ($\dot{M}$) related to the cross-sectional area (A) across which diffusion occurs as well as the thickness of the membrane (ℓ)?

2

Functional Pulmonary Anatomy

The major function of the lung is to exchange gas between the outside environment and blood. This requires an intricate structure that provides for optimal matching of blood flow and ventilation to allow efficient gas exchange with minimal energy cost. The study of respiratory physiology elucidates the many mechanisms that optimize gas exchange during health and that deteriorate in lung disease.

In the lungs, gas exchange occurs via passive diffusion along a partial pressure gradient. The barrier between gas and blood is extremely thin and large in area so that this diffusive gas exchange can take place even under severe demands such as heavy exercise.

Inhaled air passes along a branching network of progressively narrower, shorter, and more numerous airways that end in small air sacs called *alveoli*. Blood flows through an intricate network of blood vessels that eventually perfuse the very small alveolar capillaries lying on the opposite side of the alveolar wall from the air. The relative thinness (about 0.1 to 0.5 μm) of the alveolocapillary "barrier" allows for easy gas exchange.

The airway first bifurcates at the carina (located at the base of the trachea) into the left and right main stem bronchi that enter the left and right lungs, respectively (Fig. 2.1). These main bronchi separate into smaller bronchi feeding the five lobes of the human lung (upper, middle, and lower lobes on the right; upper and lower lobes on the left). The bronchi further divide into smaller bronchi feeding the segments of each lobe and, further, the lobules of each segment. The outer surface of the lung is covered with a membrane called the *visceral pleura*, while the inner surface of the chest wall is covered with a membrane termed the *parietal pleura* (Fig. 2.1). These two membranes are closely apposed to each other; the

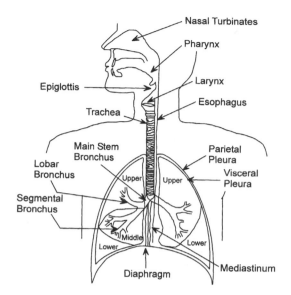

Figure 2.1. Upper airways and lobes of the human lung. The thoracic cavity is divided by the mediastinum into two major chambers that contain the right and left lungs. The right lung has three lobes (upper, middle, and lower) separated into ten segments, whereas the left lung is divided into two lobes (upper and lower) composed of nine segments. The airways are shown only through the third to fourth generations.

intervening space is termed the *pleural space*. A thin fluid layer occupies the pleural space.

Mouth, Nose, Pharynx, and Larynx

With each inspiration, air first passes through the nose and/or mouth, as shown in Figure 2.1. Turbinates, a complex structure of irregular passages in the nose, help trap inhaled particles and warm and humidify the inspired air. Whether inhaled through the nose or mouth, air reaches the pharynx, which is located at the back of the oronasal cavity above the glottis. Air then passes into the larynx, through the vocal cords, and into the trachea. During swallowing the epiglottis folds backward, totally occluding the entrance to the larynx and preventing food from entering the airways.

Airways

The tracheobronchial tree, an arrangement of branching tubes, begins at the larynx. The largest airway is the trachea, designated as generation 0. The airway tree progressively bifurcates down to the alveolar sacs (generation 23). Although the airways are not symmetrical in branching angle or size, each generation bifurcates into two daughter branches. This continues with each division, where the number of airways in a given generation is 2 raised to the power of the generation number. Thus there is 1 trachea, 2 main bronchi, 4 lobar bronchi, 16 segmental bronchi, and so forth. Each generation is progressively smaller in both diameter and length (Table 2.1). The larger conducting airways (generations 0 through 16) transport air between the outside and the gas-exchanging regions of the lungs. The smaller respiratory airways (generations 17 through 23) not only conduct air but also permit gas diffusion, which increases in significance closer to the alveoli. The branching pattern of the larger airways is somewhat irregular and asymmetrical, leading to nonuniformities in airway length and cross-sectional area (even within a given generation number).

Table 2.1. Dimensions of Adult Human Airways

GENERATION	NO. PER GENERATION	DIAMETER (cm)	LENGTH (cm)	TOTAL CROSS SECTIONAL AREA (cm^2)	TOTAL VOLUME (cm^3)
0	1	1.8	12.0	2.54	30.54
1	2	1.22	4.76	2.33	41.67
2	4	0.83	1.90	2.13	45.78
3	8	0.56	0.76	2.00	47.28
4	16	0.45	1.27	2.48	50.51
5	32	0.35	1.07	3.11	53.80
6	64	0.28	0.90	3.96	57.35
7	128	0.23	0.76	5.10	61.39
8	256	0.186	0.64	6.95	65.84
9	512	0.154	0.54	9.56	70.99
10	1,024	0.130	0.46	13.4	77.24
11	2,048	0.109	0.39	19.6	84.70
12	4,096	0.095	0.33	28.8	94.28
13	8,192	0.082	0.27	44.5	105.96
14	16,384	0.074	0.23	69.4	122.17
15	32,768	0.066	0.20	113.0	144.59
16	65,536	0.060	0.165	180.0	175.16
17	131,072	0.054	0.141	300.0	217.49
18	262,144	0.050	0.117	*	*
19	524,288	0.047	0.099	*	*
20	1,048,576	0.045	0.083	*	*
21	2,097,152	0.043	0.070	*	*
22	†				
23	†				

* Cross-sectional area and total volume increase dramatically beyond the 17th generation because of the presence of alveoli, which increase in number in these more distal airways. The acinus includes the airways and alveoli distal to the primary respiratory bronchiole.

† The dimensions of generations 22 and 23 cannot be easily listed because of the numerous alveoli attached to these airways.

Conducting Airways

Trachea

The trachea, the single airway originating at the larynx, is supported by C-shaped cartilage pieces that are joined posteriorly by tissue containing smooth muscle bands. During a forceful exhalation this tissue can invaginate into the lumen of the airways when pressure on the outside exceeds that on the inside of the trachea, thereby causing a tremendous reduction in the cross-sectional area available for gas flow (see Chapter 3). The tracheal mucosa contains columnar, ciliated epithelium and numerous mucus-secreting goblet cells (Fig. 2.2). The cilia beat in a coordinated manner, causing the mouthward movement of mucus and inhaled particles, an important mechanism for elimination of inhaled foreign particles (Fig. 2.3). This

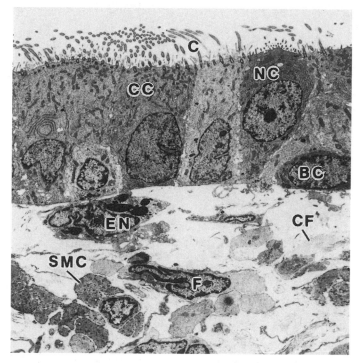

Figure 2.2. A transmission electron micrograph of a section of the conducting zone airway. The epithelium of the conducting zone is composed of different cell types. The major cell types are the columnar epithelial cell (CC) with cilia (C) and the nonciliated epithelial cell (NC). Also shown are basal cells (BC), extravascular neutrophil (EN), collagen fibrils (CF), smooth muscle cells (SMC), and fibroblasts (F). (Courtesy of Dr. D.L. Luchtel, Department of Environmental Health, University of Washington.)

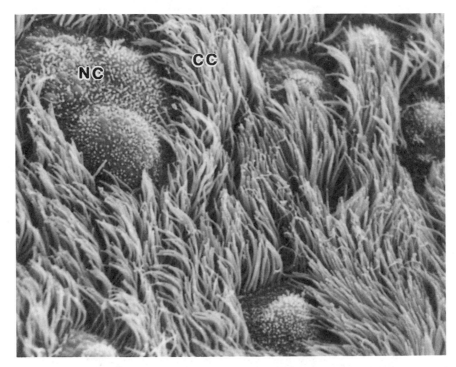

Figure 2.3. Scanning electron micrograph of the surface of a bronchus showing cilia on the ciliated epithelial cell (CC) and the nonciliated microvillous cell (NC). The coordinated movements of cilia help to move mucus and inhaled particles mouthward for elimination from the lungs. Between the patches of cilia are the microvilli on NCs. (Courtesy of Dr. D.L. Luchtel, Department of Environmental Health, University of Washington.)

system is termed the *mucociliary escalator*. Cilial beat may become ineffective under certain conditions such as anesthesia, smoking, or prolonged dry air inspiration.

Main, Lobar, and Segmental Bronchi

The trachea bifurcates asymmetrically; the right main bronchus is wider and forms a smaller angle with the long axis of the trachea. It is thus more likely to receive large inhaled particles. Main, lobar, and segmental bronchi have firm cartilaginous support in their walls, which is C shaped in the main bronchi, but takes the form of irregularly shaped, helical plates lower down. The bronchial epithelium is similar to that in the trachea, although the height of the cells gradually diminishes in the more peripheral air passages until the epithelial cells become cuboidal in the bronchioles (Table 2.2). In addition to mucous-secreting goblet cells in the bronchial

Table 2.2. Airway Structure

STRUCTURE	GENERATION NUMBER		EPITHELIAL CELL TYPE	CILIATED EPITHELIUM	CARTILAGE	GOBLET CELLS	SMOOTH MUSCLE	ALVEOLI
Trachea	0	⎫	Columnar	++*	+++	++	++	0
Bronchi	1–4	⎬ Conducting zone		++	++	++	++	0
Small bronchi	5–11	⎭	↓	+	+	+	+++	0
Bronchioles	12–16			+	0	+/0	+	0
Respiratory bronchioles	17–19	⎫ Respiratory zone	Cuboidal	0	0	0	+	+
Alveolar ducts	20–22	⎭	↓	0	0	0	+	++
Alveolar sacs	23		Squamous	0	0	0	0	+++

* The symbols zero, plus, etc. indicate the relative number of specific constituents, from nonpresent (zero) to numerous (+++).

epithelium, there is also present submucosal glands that have ducts going to the bronchial surface and release mucus onto the surface of the bronchial epithelium. Total cross-sectional area of the respiratory tract decreases for the first three generations and is minimal at the third generation (Table 2.1).

Small Bronchi

The small bronchi extend through about seven generations (from about airway generations 5 to 11), and their diameter progressively falls from 3.5 to 1 mm. Because their number doubles with each generation, the total cross-sectional area increases markedly with each generation. This substantially reduces airway resistance in the smaller airways.

Down to the level of the smallest bronchi, air passages lie close to branches of the pulmonary artery in a sheath also containing pulmonary lymphatics. The pressure within this sheath is low so that when edema occurs fluid accumulates here at an early stage (see Chapter 5). The decrease in airway size may decrease ventilation to the lung region distal to the airway narrowing.

Increased mucus production in diseases such as asthma and chronic bronchitis results in a narrowing of the airway luminal size. The consequent increase in airway resistance can result in a significant limitation in airflow and thereby the ability of the patient to ventilate adequately.

no cartilage
Bronchioles   *lung*

A significant transition occurs around the 11th generation where the average airway diameter is about 1 mm. Cartilage disappears from the bronchial wall below this level, and structural rigidity ceases to be a factor in maintaining patency. Beyond generation 11, the airways are directly embedded in the lung parenchyma, and elastic recoil holds the air passages open. Therefore, the size of the airways below the 11th generation is influenced mainly by lung volume. The distending forces holding the airways open are stronger at higher lung volumes. Increased lung volume thus expands bronchiole size and decreases airway resistance, whereas decreased lung volume may lead to airway closure, particularly in the more dependent* regions of the lungs (see Chapter 3). Normally humans sigh (a single, large inhaled breath) once every few minutes, which helps to expand those regions that may have closed airways.

At the bronchiole level there is a reduction in the number of ciliated epithelial cells as the epithelium becomes progressively cuboidal. There is also a decrease in mucus-secreting goblet cells.

---

*The lower part of the lung is termed "dependent" because it is thought of as being suspended from the upper part of the lung.

In succeeding generations, the number of bronchioles increases far more rapidly than the diameter diminishes. Therefore, the total cross-sectional area increases until, in the terminal bronchioles, it is about 30 times the area at the level of the main stem bronchi. The flow resistance of the smaller air passages is only about one-tenth of that of the whole airway system (see Chapter 3).

The walls of the bronchioles are composed of helical muscular bands of smooth muscle cells. In asthma, contraction of the muscle bands in response to an antigen decreases airway diameter and wrinkles the mucosa into longitudinal folds. This increases airflow resistance and may result in airway obstruction.

Down to the level of the terminal bronchioles (the last-order bronchiole just before the appearance of alveoli in the walls of the airways), the air passages derive their nutrition from the bronchial circulation and are thus influenced by systemic arterial blood gas levels. Beyond this point the smaller air passages rely on the pulmonary circulation for their nutrition. In the presence of diseases obstructing the pulmonary circulation to a region, however, the bronchial circulation can hypertrophy and become responsible for the nutrition of the small airways.

Respiratory Airways

Respiratory Bronchioles

The functions of the air passages down to the terminal bronchioles are primarily air conduction, humidification, and warming. In the respiratory bronchioles a gradual transition in function from conduction to gas exchange occurs. In the three generations of respiratory bronchioles, there is a progressive increase in the number of alveoli (gas-exchange air sacs) in their walls (Fig. 2.4). The epithelium is cuboidal between the mouths of the alveoli in the earlier generations of respiratory bronchioles but becomes progressively flatter until it is entirely alveolar epithelium (squamous) within the alveolar ducts. Like the conducting bronchioles, respiratory bronchioles are embedded in lung parenchyma. They have a well-marked muscle layer, however, with bands that loop around the opening of the alveolar ducts and the mouths of the alveoli.

The *terminal respiratory unit,* also known at the *pulmonary acinus,* is defined as the lung region supplied by a first-order respiratory bronchiole. According to this definition, there are about 130,000 terminal units—each with a diameter of about 3.5 mm and containing about 2000 alveoli, each of these being small enough for gases to be well mixed by diffusion.

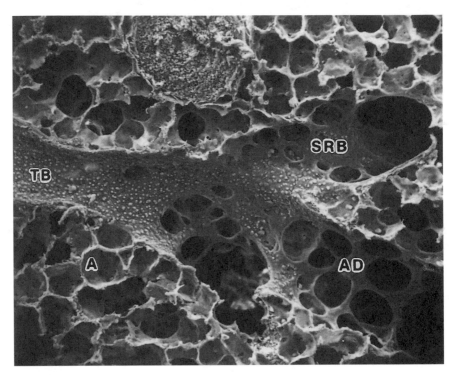

Figure 2.4. Scanning electron micrograph of a terminal bronchiole (TB) transitioning to alveolar ducts (AD) through very short respiratory bronchioles (SRB). The conduction function is apparent from the tubular shape. The respiratory function is apparent from the large number of alveoli (A) coming off the wall of the respiratory bronchiole. (Courtesy of Dr. B.K. Ross, Department of Anesthesiology, University of Washington.)

Alveolar Ducts

Alveolar ducts arise from the respiratory bronchiole. The alveolar duct has no walls other than alveoli that are arranged in a cylindrical pattern of rings (Fig. 2.5). Gas transport within the alveolar ducts is accomplished primarily by diffusion.

Alveoli

The alveoli (Fig. 2.6) are the last generation of the air passages. The walls of the alveoli are very thin (0.1 to 0.2 μm), and this provides for easy exchange of gases between the alveolar air and blood in the pulmonary capillaries (see Fig. 2.8, later). Alveoli arise from airway generations 17 through 23. There are approximately 300 million alveoli in the human lung, providing a very large surface area (approximately 70 m^2) for gas exchange. The efficiency of this exchange is discussed in Chapter 7.

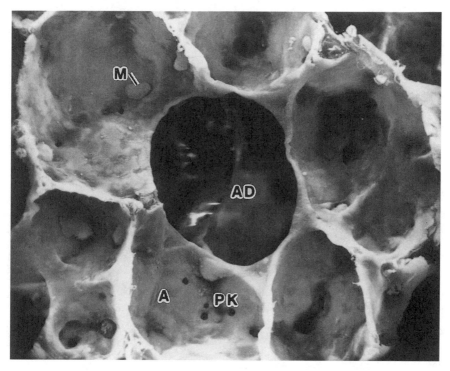

Figure 2.5. Scanning electron micrograph of an alveolar duct (AD). Looking down the axis of the duct, a ring of alveoli (A) is evident. Additional alveoli are located behind the alveoli shown in the view. In some of the alveoli, pores of Kohn (PK) and alveolar macrophages (M) can be seen. (Courtesy of Dr. B.K. Ross, Department of Anesthesiology, University of Washington.)

Blood Vessels

Pulmonary Circulation

The pulmonary circulation carries the entire cardiac output of blood from the right ventricle to the lungs for gas exchange. The main pulmonary artery divides into two smaller muscular arteries that go to the right and left lungs. These vessels continue to divide into smaller arterioles that gradually decrease in amount of smooth muscle until practically no muscle exists in the very small arterioles. The branching set of vessels eventually reaches the pulmonary capillaries. Arterial vessels are distributed along airways all the way to the alveoli. Pulmonary capillaries (about 5 to 7 µm in radius) track along the alveolar walls, passing several alveoli

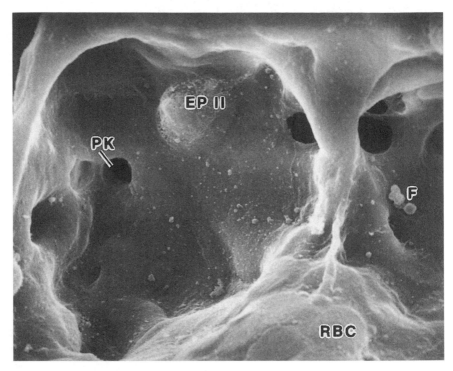

Figure 2.6. Scanning electron micrograph of an alveolus showing the presence in the alveolar wall of an alveolar epithelial type II cell (EP II). Several pores of Kohn (PK) are shown, providing connections between adjacent alveoli. An outline of an intravascular red blood cell (RBC) shows through the alveolar wall. Fragments (F) of cellular material created by the fixation process are evident. (Courtesy of Dr. B.K. Ross, Department of Anesthesiology, University of Washington.)

before the blood is collected in the venous system. The venules gradually join into larger vessels and eventually reach pulmonary veins that connect directly to the left atrium.

Pulmonary arteries are more compliant than systemic arteries because they are much thinner and have proportionately more elastic tissue in their walls. The walls of the arterioles (100 μm diameter and smaller) are so thin, in contrast to their systemic counterparts, that fluid and gas can move across them (see Chapter 5). They are narrow, and their intravascular pressure is low; thus they need very few smooth muscle fibers to regulate flow.

Pulmonary capillaries form a continuous network in the alveolar walls throughout a lobe. When distended by intravascular pressure, they are so numerous that blood flows almost as an unbroken sheet between the airspaces (Fig. 2.7). "Sheet flow" reduces vascular resistance and optimizes gas exchange. When the pressure difference between the inside and outside of the vessels (transmural pressure) is low, some of the capillary segments are closed, but they are easily opened and recruited into the pulmonary vascular bed by a transmural pressure increase. The open capillaries distend when their transmural pressure rises, as when cardiac output increases. It takes many seconds for a red cell to flow from the pulmonary artery to the vein at the periphery (top or bottom) of the lung, but only a fraction of a second in central regions of the lower lobe. The average transit time (time available for gas exchange) through the vessels is calculated to be about 0.75 seconds at rest.

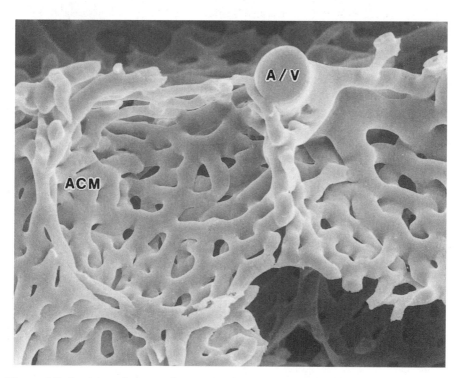

Figure 2.7. Scanning electron micrograph of a cast of the alveolar capillary bed meshwork (ACM). The capillary network around each alveolus forms a nearly continuous sheet of blood. Adjacent alveoli share a single capillary mesh in their common wall. It is likely that blood traverses several alveoli in passing from the arteriole to the venule. The large vessel (A/V) at the top is either an arteriole or a venule. (From Guntheroth WG et al. Pulmonary microcirculation: Tubules rather than sheet and post. *J Appl Physiol* 53:510–515, 1982.)

Bronchial Circulation

The bronchial circulation, part of the systemic circulation, provides oxygenated blood to the pulmonary airway tissue. The bronchial arteries originate from the intercostal arteries and the descending thoracic aorta. The arterioles and capillaries are interspersed within the airway wall down to the terminal bronchioles. The bronchial circulation provides perfusion to the pleura for nutrition of that tissue. There are extensive small vessel anastomoses (communications) between the bronchial vessels and the pulmonary vasculature.

The bronchial circulation drains in two ways. The veins from larger airways empty via the systemic veins into the azygos vein and into the right atrium. Much of the drainage from the intrapulmonary bronchial circulation goes into the pulmonary circulation (either pre- or post capillary) and returns via the pulmonary veins to the left heart. This blood adds deoxygenated blood to the systemic arterial circulation and is a source of anatomical shunt. The total anatomical shunt is about 2% to 5% of cardiac output (see Chapter 7). The bronchial circulation provides the water necessary to humidify the inspired air as it passes through the airways. It is also the source of highly soluble gases, such as ethyl alcohol, that exchange with inspired air entirely within the airways rather than in the alveoli, where O_2 and CO_2 are exchanged.

Lymphatics

Pulmonary lymphatic circulation carries fluid from the interstitial space in the alveoli back to the systemic circulation. The lymphatics also originate around small airways and blood vessels and at the pleural surface. The main lymphatic channels are located along the bronchial tree. Lymph nodes are located along these main channels and serve to filter the lymph before it enters the circulatory system. Lymph flows through the right lymphatic duct and left thoracic duct into the innominate vein in the upper chest. The total flow from the lungs is normally less than 0.5 ml · min^{-1} but can increase up to tenfold with pulmonary edema. When edema fluid production in the alveolar spaces becomes large enough to exceed the capacity of the lymphatics, severe edema results. Interstitial fluid pressure then rises high enough to disrupt the alveolar epithelial integrity, resulting in alveolar edema.

Alveoli and Alveolocapillary Membrane

Alveoli

The alveoli are packed closely together. Because they share walls with abutting alveoli, the shape of an alveolus is not truly spherical but can be described as an irregular polyhedron with one face cut off at its entrance. It is estimated that there are about 300 million alveoli in adult human lungs, each with an average diameter of about 300 μm at 75% of maximum lung volume. In the intact lung there is a gradient in alveolar size; the alveoli at the top of the lung are the largest, while those at the bases are the smallest. This gradient results from the effects of gravity; more lung tissue (and blood) pulls down on the upper part of the lung, causing greater distention of the upper alveoli. This distribution varies with position or changes in lung volume.

The alveolar walls have small holes (pores of Kohn) about 10 to 15 μm in diameter that connect the gas spaces of adjacent alveoli (Fig. 2.6). These pores may allow mixing of gas between adjacent alveoli. This idea has been questioned, however, because there could be a thin liquid film covering these pores in the *in vivo* situation. With age or development of emphysema, there is a breakdown of alveolar walls, and more and larger openings are present.

Alveolocapillary Membrane

Three major cell types are found in the alveoli. Type I, or squamous alveolar epithelial, cells cover most of the alveolar surface, and these cells have few cytoplasmic organelles. From the nucleus the cytoplasm extends out in broad, thin plates a fraction of a micron thick that constitute the main cellular lining of the alveoli (Fig. 2.8). The type II, or granular alveolar cell, is roughly spherical with many microvilli on its surface. It contains many cellular organelles, including large numbers of osmiophilic granules that show a layered structure called *lamellar bodies*. Type II cells are not surface-covering cells like type I cells; they do not send out cytoplasmic extensions to cover the alveolar surface. The alveolar–air interface has a surface lining layer of a lipoprotein, the pulmonary surfactant, which keeps the surface tension at the air–surface interface low, helping to prevent alveolar collapse (see Chapter 3). Type II cells are the source of this surfactant. Finally, the third major cell type is the alveolar macrophage, this call type lies on top of the alveolar lining provided by the type I cells. The macrophages move freely over the surface of the alveoli and phagocytose any extraneous material that enters the alveoli, including bacteria and particulates. Macrophages are cleared via the airways and lymphatics.

The layer separating blood and air is the alveolocapillary barrier, across which gases diffuse during the gas exchange process (Fig. 2.8). It consists of the surfactant lining layer, the aqueous hypophase, a thin layer of cytoplasm of type I cells, the interstitium, and the thin endothelial cell lining of the capillary (Fig. 2.8). In most areas the basement membranes of the squamous alveolar epithelial cells and the endothelial cells are fused. In other regions the basement membranes are separated, and elastic fibers and collagen fibers may be seen in the interstitial space. To promote gas exchange, this alveolocapillary barrier must be as thin as possible and

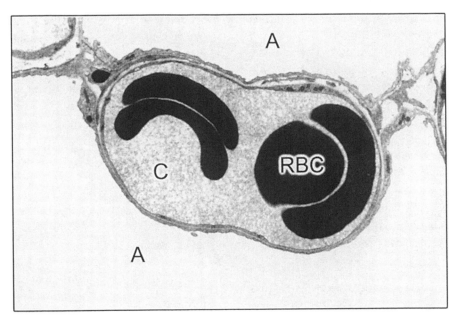

A

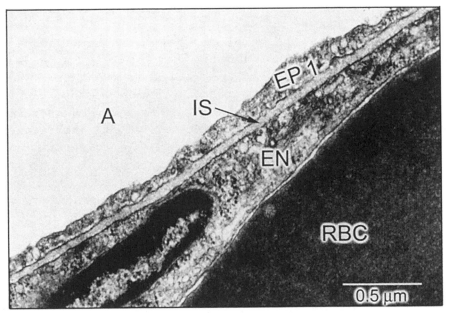

B

the surface area as large as possible. The mean thickness of the diffusion barrier between alveolar gas and the red cell is only on average about 0.5 µm, providing a minimal diffusion distance for O_2 and CO_2.

Respiratory Muscles

The muscles of respiration serve to change the pleural pressure; this leads to differences between the pressure within the gas phase of the alveoli and the pressure outside the body. These differences result in air flow. Muscles of respiration have no inherent rhythm and rely on the central respiratory control system (see Chapter 8) for their rhythmic activation.

There are a number of important diseases that can restrict or eliminate the functioning of the respiratory muscles. These are broadly classified as neuromuscular diseases and include diseases involving the spinal cord, motor nerves, synaptic transmission at the neuromuscular junction, or the muscles themselves. Failure of the respiratory muscles and resultant death as a consequence of progression of neuromuscular diseases such as amyotrophic lateral sclerosis, poliomyelitis, and myasthenia gravis are examples illustrating the paramount importance of the respiratory muscles.

Muscles of Inspiration

Inspiration is an active process and can occur only when the inspiratory muscles contract (in the absence of any external ventilation system). The primary inspiratory muscle is the diaphragm; this is a large, dome-shaped sheet of muscle separating the abdominal and thoracic cavities (Fig. 2.9A). It is anchored around the circumference of the lower thoracic cage and also to the vertebral column. It bulges up

---

Figure 2.8. Transmission electron micrographs of the alveolocapillary barrier. **A** Low-power electron micrograph of transverse section of a pulmonary capillary (C) containing red blood cells (RBCs). Note that the alveolar (A) gas space is separated from the plasma and the RBCs by a thin alveolocapillary barrier. (From Velazquez M et al. PET evaluation of pulmonary vascular permeability: A structure–function correlation. *J Appl Physiol* 70: 2206–2216, 1991.) **B** High-power electron micrograph of the alveolocapillary barrier. The cellular elements of the alveolocapillary barrier are thin, consisting of type I alveolar epithelia cells (EP 1) and capillary endothelial cells (EN) that are separated by a narrow interstitial space (IS). The surfactant lining layer, which normally overlies the alveolar epithelial cells and is part of the alveolocapillary barrier, is not evident in this micrograph. (Courtesy of Dr. D.L. Luchtel, Department of Environmental Health, University of Washington.)

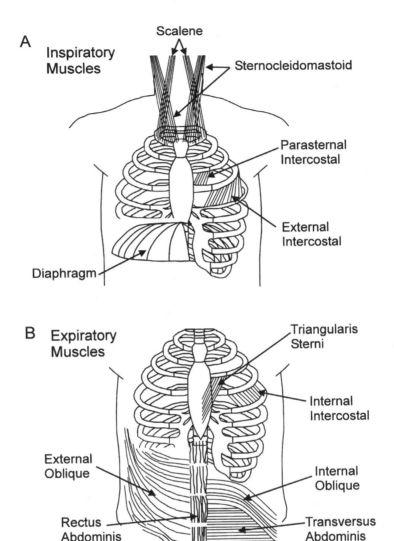

Figure 2.9. The muscles of respiration. During inspiration **(A)**, the diaphragm moves downward, and the external intercostals and parasternal intercostals pull the ribs upward and outward. The muscles in the neck, scalene, and sternocleidomastoid act to elevate the thorax and also to stabilize the upper ribs. During passive expiration, the inspiratory muscles relax, and the compliance of the chest wall returns the ribs to their relaxed position, thereby expelling air. During forced expiration **(B)**, the internal intercostals can pull the ribs downward and inward; the triangularis sterni muscles when activated pull the ribs to which they are attached downward. There are four sets of expiratory abdominal muscles, external oblique, rectus abdominis, internal oblique, and transversus abdominis. These muscles when activated pull the lower ribs downward and compress the abdomen. For clarity in this figure, each representative rib cage muscle is shown within only one rib interspace; in reality these muscles are in multiple rib interspaces.

toward the thoracic cavity. Contraction of the diaphragm pulls down the central part, acting like a piston to increase the volume of the thoracic cavity. The descent of the diaphragm results in an increase in intraabdominal pressure. This pressure increase, coupled with the dome shape of the diaphragm, causes expansion of the lower rib cage.

The external intercostal muscles (inspiratory muscles) are located between adjacent bony (interosseous) ribs and are innervated by the intercostal nerves. These muscles are arranged so that contraction results in upward and outward movement of the ribs. The ribs pivot from the vertebral column in a bucket-handle fashion so that external intercostal muscle contraction increases the cross-sectional area of the thoracic cavity. Between the cartilagenous (interchondral) portions of each of the upper ribs the intercostal muscles are in a single layer. These intercostals are called the *parasternal intercostal muscles*. The parasternals are inspiratory muscles and are active even in quiet breathing.

Other respiratory muscles help to enhance the volume-increasing motion during inspiration. Contraction of the scalene muscles, by pulling up on the first two ribs, functions to elevate the thorax. These muscles are active even in quiet breathing and are further activated during increased ventilation. The sternocleidomastoid muscles are not active during quiet breathing but are activated during increased ventilation when they function, as do the scalene muscles, to elevate the thorax.

Muscles of Expiration

Normally expiration is passive. Airflow is accomplished by relaxation of the inspiratory muscles, and flow results from the stored elastic energy of the expanded thorax. During increased ventilation or forced exhalation, however, other muscles are activated (Fig. 2.9B). The internal intercostal muscles (expiratory muscles) are located between adjacent interosseous ribs. Contraction of these muscles lowers the ribs, moving them downward and inward, and stiffens the intercostal spaces. Another important expiratory muscle of the rib cage is the triangularis sterni. The triangularis sterni muscles are attached between the inner side of the sternum and the interchondral portions of the upper ribs. When activated, their function is to pull downward the ribs to which they are attached. This muscle group is not active in quiet breathing but becomes activated when expiratory muscles are recruited. The expiratory abdominal muscles are made up of four unique muscle layers that are active during expiration; these are the external oblique, rectus abdominis, internal oblique, and transversus abdominis. Contraction of these muscles lowers the bottom ribs and increases intraabdominal pressure, forcing the diaphragm upward.

The diaphragm is also active to a limited degree early in the expiratory phase.

It can serve as a brake on expiration and causes a smoother and less abrupt expiration. Later in expiration the diaphragm relaxes completely.

Further Reading

1. Decramer M. The respiratory muscles. In: Fishman A P, editor. *Pulmonary Diseases and Disorders,* 3rd ed. New York: McGraw-Hill, 1998, pp 63–71.
2. Horsfield, K. Morphometry of airways. In: Macklem P T, Mead J, editors. *Handbook of Physiology.* Section 3, *The Respiratory System*, vol III, *Mechanics of Breathing,* part 1. Bethesda, MD: American Physiological Society, 1986, pp 75–88.
3. Proctor D F. Form and function of the upper airways and larynx. In: Macklem P T, Mead J, editors. *Handbook of Physiology.* Section 3, *The Respiratory System*, vol III, *Mechanics of Breathing,* part 1. Bethesda, MD: American Physiological Society, 1986, pp 63–74.
4. Weibel, E R, Taylor, C R. Functional design of the human lung for gas exchange. In: Fishman A P, editor. *Pulmonary Diseases and Disorders,* 3rd ed. New York: McGraw-Hill, 1998, pp 21–61.

Study Questions

2.1. How do the upper airways help to protect the delicate alveolar tissues?

2.2. Which airway generation numbers benefit from cartilage as a means of structural support?

2.3. In which airway generations are ciliated epithelial cells present to assist in the mouthward transfer of mucus?

2.4. Where does the transition occur between the conducting terminal bronchioles and the respiratory bronchioles?

2.5. Explain the "sheet flow" concept of alveolar blood flow.

2.6. Describe the role and pathway of bronchial circulation.

2.7. Describe the muscles of inspiration and of expiration.

3

Mechanics of Ventilation

Movement of air between the environment and the alveoli is governed by mechanical properties of the lungs and chest wall and by characteristics of air flow in the airways. These mechanical factors are fundamental to mammalian respiration and to an understanding of the impact of stress and/or disease on respiration. In fact, many pulmonary function tests designed to quantitate disease measure airflow and volume properties of the lung.

Static Properties

Lung volume is divided into several overlapping components (Fig. 3.1), each of which varies from individual to individual and depends on age and body size; larger individuals have larger lung volumes. Tidal volume (V_T) is the volume of the air that moves in and out in a single breath. Normally, a person begins inhalation of V_T from functional residual capacity (FRC), the volume of gas within the lungs after total relaxation of all respiratory muscles.

When one inhales to a maximum volume, total lung capacity (TLC) is limited by the distensibility of both the lungs and the chest wall as well as the amount of additional force the inspiratory muscles can exert. The maximum volume that can be exhaled from TLC is the vital capacity (VC). The volume remaining in the lungs after a complete exhalation is residual volume (RV), which is determined by mechanical limitations of the chest wall and diaphragm, airway closure (particularly in older individuals and those with lung disease), and the amount of additional force the expiratory muscles can exert.

The volume that can be inhaled from FRC is the inspiratory capacity (IC) and is equal to TLC minus FRC. The volume available to inhale after a normal V_T

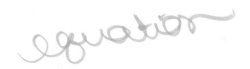

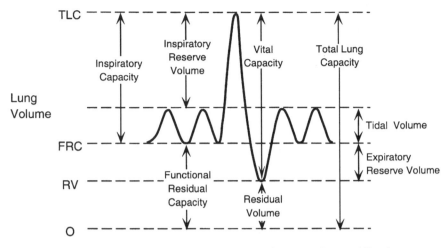

Figure 3.1. Spirometry of the lungs shows various static lung volumes. All volumes except those including residual volume can be measured with a spirometer.

inhalation is inspiratory reserve volume (IRV), which is equal to TLC minus FRC minus V_T. Likewise, the maximal volume that can be exhaled after a relaxed exhalation is expiratory reserve volume (ERV), equal to FRC minus RV.

The convention is to express the various volumes that cannot be broken down into smaller components as a "volume." Any volume that is a combination of other volumes is called a "capacity." These volumes and capacities are not anatomically distinct regions, but are distributed throughout the lungs.

All of the volumes that are exhaled from the mouth can be measured with a spirometer, which measures either volume or flow and time during either inspiration or expiration. The expired flow signal can be electronically integrated to provide volume. The expired volume signal can be differentiated to provide flow.

Two methods are available to measure those volumes or capacities that include RV, the volume that cannot be exhaled. Inert gas dilution uses the conservation of mass principle (Chapter 1). If a subject (having no helium in the lungs) rebreathes from a bag containing an initial helium concentration (F_{1He}), the helium will dilute into the combined bag and lung volume after several rebreathed breaths giving a lower helium concentration (F_{2He}). After equilibration, the FRC can be calculated using the following relationship:

$$FRC = V_{bag}\left(\frac{F_{1He} - F_{2He}}{F_{2He}}\right) \qquad (3.1)$$

where V_{bag} is the initial volume of the rebreathing bag.

A second method uses a body plethysmograph (body box). The subject sits within the box and breaths against a closed valve. This method uses the principle of Boyle's law ($P_1V_1 = P_2V_2$) and compares the change in pressure within the lung to the change in pressure outside the body (but within the box). The lung volume is proportional to the ratio of the change of pressure within the box to the change of pressure within the lung. The latter pressure is measured within the mouth of the subject, when the subject's mouth and nasal passages are closed. For greater detail on the application of these methods for measuring FRC, see Hughes and Pride (1999).

Measurement of the volumes and capacities provides the basis for assessing mechanical lung function and a means for quantifying the effects of lung disease.

The Lung–Chest Wall System

Together, the lung and chest wall contribute to the elastic properties of the respiratory system. The chest wall component also includes the diaphragm and part of the abdominal wall. Under normal circumstances, the outer surface of the lungs (visceral pleura) and the inner surface of the chest wall (parietal pleura) are in intimate contact, held together by the negative intrapleural pressure. The intermolecular forces of the pleural fluid hold the two together like a liquid film does between two pieces of glass. The two pieces of glass can slide easily relative to each other, but it is difficult to pull them apart without sliding.

Elastic Structures

The recoil tendency of a spring can be expressed in terms of an unstressed or resting length and a length–tension relationship. Similarly, for expandable volumetric structures, the relevant properties are the unstressed volume and the pressure–volume relationship. *Distending pressure is* expressed as the difference between the pressures inside and outside the structure ($P_{in} - P_{out}$). The pressure difference is also called the *recoil pressure*, reflecting the tendency of the structure to return to its unstressed volume (where transmural distending or recoil pressure is zero). A positive recoil pressure indicates a tendency to get smaller. A structure distorted to a volume below its unstressed volume will have a negative recoil pressure, or a tendency to get larger.

Elastic Properties of the Lung

The elastic properties of the lung can be likened to those of a balloon. While inflated, there is a tendency to recoil (or collapse) to a smaller unstressed volume. To keep the lung inflated, a distending pressure difference is required between the alveolar pressure (P_A) and the intrapleural pressure (P_{pl}) surrounding the lung. This distending force is provided by the elastic properties of the chest wall and the respiratory muscles. The elastic properties of the lung can be expressed by plotting lung volume against the distending (or recoil) pressure (Fig. 3.2). These elastic properties are the same irrespective of the mode of ventilation (i.e., spontaneous ventilation, which exerts a negative intrapleural pressure, or mechanical ventilation, which exerts a positive pressure at the mouth). In addition, the pressure–volume curve is independent of the magnitude or direction of airflow.

The slope of this pressure–volume curve represents the ease of distention of the lungs (L). This slope is termed the *compliance* (C):

$$C_L = \frac{\Delta V}{\Delta P} \tag{3.2}$$

expressed as $l \cdot cm\ H_2O^{-1}$. The compliance depends on lung volume and decreases as the lungs approach the maximum limit of distention at TLC. At this point, elastin fibers within the lung parenchyma are near the limits of their ability to stretch. Compliance is usually measured in the normal tidal breathing range near FRC.

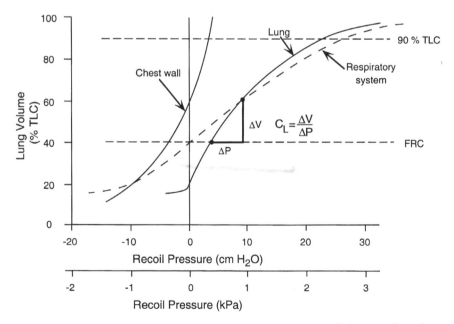

Figure 3.2. Static pressure–volume relationships for the chest wall, lung, and respiratory system. These "relaxation" curves, obtained with all of the respiratory muscles relaxed, describe the passive mechanical properties of the respiratory system.

Because the compliance is expressed in absolute volume terms, it is dependent on lung size. In comparing the relative ability of lung tissue to stretch, it is helpful to normalize by lung volume. The specific lung compliance (C_{sp}) is derived by dividing the lung compliance by the lung volume (V_L) at which it is measured (most often, FRC):

$$C_{sp} = \frac{C_L}{V_L} \tag{3.3}$$

The specific lung compliances of a child and an adult may be similar even though their absolute compliances are quite different.

Elastic Properties of the Chest Wall

The chest wall has a larger unstressed volume than the lungs and resists deformation as the volume is changed in either direction from this unstressed volume. A pressure–volume curve for the chest wall is included in Figure 3.2. In this case, the recoil pressure refers to the pressure difference across the chest wall (pleural pressure minus atmospheric pressure [$P_{pl} - P_{atm}$]). This relaxation curve applies only when respiratory muscles are completely relaxed. As the chest wall expands, compliance of the lungs becomes very small, limiting further expansion of the respiratory system. Similarly, decreasing lung volume is eventually limited because of distortion of the chest wall and a very low chest wall compliance. In older individuals airway closure may decrease the lung compliance; this limits the decrease in lung volume before reaching the low chest wall compliance and will result in a higher residual volume. In the normal tidal breathing range, compliance of the chest wall is similar to that of the lungs, and each is about twice the compliance of the total respiratory system.

Lung and Chest Wall: The Respiratory System

Normally the lungs and chest wall expand together. Because there is no air in the pleural space, the volume of gas within the chest wall is identical to the volume of gas within the lungs. Pleural fluid serves to lubricate the movement of the lung and chest wall relative to each other. The pleural fluid is produced by filtration from the parietal pleural capillaries (because of the higher pressure of the systemic circulation), circulates within the pleural space, and is reabsorbed by the visceral pleural capillaries. The circulation of pleural liquid in the pleural space is governed by downward flow due to gravity, upward flow along lobar margins, and transverse flow caused by the movements of the pleural surfaces caused by breathing.

Recoil pressure for the respiratory system ($P_A - P_{atm}$) is equal to the sum of recoil pressure for the lungs ($P_A - P_{pl}$) and for the chest wall ($P_{pl} - P_{atm}$). This relationship is expressed graphically in Figure 3.2, which shows the pressure–volume curve of the respiratory system as the sum (on the pressure axis) of the pressure–volume curve for the lungs and the pressure–volume curve of the chest wall. Note that the slope of the respiratory system curve at any given volume is less than the slope for either the chest wall or lungs. Greater pressure is needed to distend the lungs and chest wall together by a given volume than it does for either separately.

The force of the respiratory muscles is not displayed in the relaxation curves of Figure 3.2, which describe the elastic properties of the lungs and chest wall alone or together. If a person were to inhale to a given volume, place the mouth on a pressure manometer, and relax the respiratory muscles, the pressure obtained would be equal to that shown on the relaxation curve of the respiratory system in Figure 3.2.

Compliance for the respiratory system (C_T) is lower than that for either the lungs or chest wall (C_{CW}). These compliances are related to one another by the following expression:

$$\frac{1}{C_T} = \frac{1}{C_L} + \frac{1}{C_{CW}} \tag{3.4}$$

At FRC, the lung is above its unstressed volume (volume assumed by the lung with a transpulmonary pressure of zero), while the chest wall is below its own unstressed volume. Also, at FRC the outward negative recoil force of the chest wall is exactly counterbalanced by the inward positive recoil force of the lungs.

Any disease process that alters the compliance of the lung or the chest wall or both will change the pressure–volume curve and alter the recoil forces, which change the FRC as well as other lung volumes. Fibrosis is a disease that decreases lung compliance, and scoliosis is a disease that decreases chest wall compliance through its effect on the spine. Also, extensive burns to the thorax decrease compliance of the chest wall.

It is important to recognize that pressure–volume characteristics of the lungs and chest wall are not altered by airflow itself. At a given lung volume, the lung compliance during a breath-hold is identical to that during either inspiration or expiration.

Events of the Respiratory Cycle

Ventilation occurs when active muscle force is applied to the relaxed respiratory system. Relaxation of the muscle force allows passive relaxation of the respiratory system back toward FRC. Figure 3.3 shows the events of the normal respiratory cycle. At FRC the recoil pressures of the lungs and of the chest wall are equal and opposite. Addition of an outward force of inspiratory muscles (Fig. 3.3B; 27 cm H_2O is used because that amount is appropriate to get the lung to a volume of 90% TLC [see Fig. 3.2]) added to the normal recoil of the respiratory system creates an alveolar pressure that is negative with respect to atmospheric pressure. With an open glottis, air flows down the pressure gradient, causing an increase in lung volume. Flow continues to increase lung volume until the sum of recoil forces of the lungs plus the chest wall offset the muscle force, resulting in an alveolar pressure of zero (relative to atmospheric pressure) (Fig. 3.3C).

A normal exhalation is initiated by relaxation of the inspiratory respiratory muscles and elimination of the outward muscle force (Fig. 3.3D). The positive recoil pressure of the respiratory system then results in an alveolar pressure that

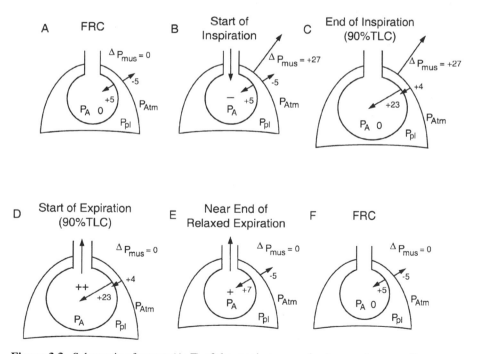

Figure 3.3. Schematic of events (A–F) of the respiratory cycle. Arrows show recoil pressure as in Figure 3.2. Pressures and flows are shown throughout the respiratory cycle.

exceeds atmospheric pressure, causing expiratory gas flow. Flow continues (Fig. 3.3E) until the lung volume is reduced to FRC (Fig. 3.3F), where the recoil pressure of the respiratory system is zero. At this point, expiratory flow ceases because alveolar pressure equals atmospheric pressure.

Normal respiration consists of an activation of inspiratory muscles during inspiration and a near complete relaxation of respiratory muscles during exhalation. Activation of expiratory muscles during exhalation can also be employed in a conscious effort to increase expiratory flow rate. In addition, activation of inspiratory muscles during exhalation can be used to retard expiratory flow rate. Both inspiratory and expiratory flow rates can be modulated with partial glottal constriction.

Expansion of Lung and Chest Wall

During breathing, the lung and chest wall change volume together despite their differing mechanical properties. The chest wall includes ribs, muscle, and other tissues, along with the diaphragm. During expansion, the constraints of the ribs' interconnections and the diaphragm contraction result in a change in shape of the chest wall that is complex in nature. The lung parenchyma is a combination of elastic and nonelastic fibers that result in lung expansion that is relatively uniform at the gross level, but distinctly non-uniform at the microscopic level. The expansion of the lung parenchyma during inspiration is constrained by the chest wall and its expansion properties, resulting in distortion of lung expansion and subtle distortions in local ventilation (due to parenchymal volume changes).

Maximal Respiratory Muscle Effort

Maximal inspiratory and expiratory pressures are governed by muscular limits and geometric constraints. Figure 3.4 shows the maximum pressures that the respiratory system can develop with maximal muscular effort. If one inhales to TLC, closes the glottis, and attempts to exhale with maximum effort (Valsalva maneuver), the pressure developed in the alveolar space will be approximately 150 cm H_2O, or about 15% of one atmosphere (1000 cm H_2O). During this maneuver, lung volume decreases slightly due to some gas compression (15%). If this experiment is done at a lower lung volume, the maximal expiratory pressure developed will be lower due to a decreased efficiency of the arrangement of the respiratory muscles and chest wall at lung volumes lower than TLC. This continues down to a zero maximal expiratory effort if the maneuver is performed at RV. If a maximal inspiratory effort against a closed glottis is performed at RV (Mueller maneuver), maximal inspiratory pressure will reach about 100 cm H_2O with a slight increase in lung volume (10%) due to gas expansion. Similarly, maximal inspiratory pressure decreases in

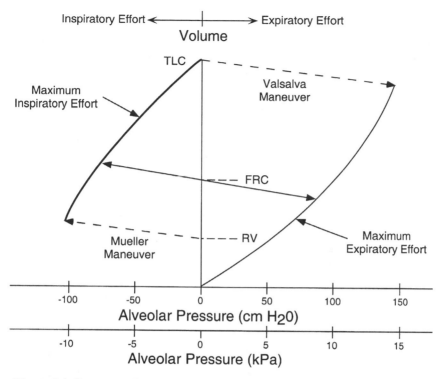

Figure 3.4. Pressure–volume curves of the respiratory system, obtained with maximal respiratory effort, demonstrate the maximum forces that can be generated by the chest wall, diaphragm, and abdominal muscles.

magnitude as lung volume increases. A maximum inspiratory effort at TLC will yield a pressure of zero.

Surface Tension

The alveolar surface is the largest epithelial surface area in the body exposed to the environment. The liquid surface presents an important protective barrier. In liquid the closeness of adjacent molecules results in large intermolecular attractive (van der Waals) forces that serve to stabilize the liquid. In the lungs the liquid–air surface produces an inequality in forces that are strong on the liquid side but very weak on the air side because of the greater distances between molecules in the gas phase. This creates a substantial surface tension that helps to sustain the integrity of the surface. The effect of surface tension is to "cause" the surface to maintain as small an area as possible. In alveoli the result is a spherical curved liquid lining layer that tends to be pulled inward toward the center of curvature of the alveolus. As a result, a greater pressure is required to expand a lung than would be the case without the presence of the alveolar liquid lining layer.

The spherical surface of the alveolar liquid lining behaves in a manner similar to a soap bubble. A bubble has two surfaces (inner and outer) that exert an inward force that creates a greater pressure inside than outside the bubble. The pressure difference caused by the curved alveolar surface can be determined from *Laplace's law*:

$$\Delta P = \frac{2\gamma}{r} \tag{3.5}$$

for single surface alveolar fluid, and

$$\Delta P = \frac{4\gamma}{r} \tag{3.6}$$

for a two surface (inside and outside) bubble, where ΔP is the pressure difference across the surface, γ is the surface tension, and r is the radius of curvature of the surface.

A consequence of the large number of interconnected alveoli with curved surface linings is the potential collapse of these alveoli into one giant alveolus. Figure 3.5 shows two bubbles connected to one another through a tube. Because of surface tension, the pressure inside the smaller bubble (with a smaller radius of curvature) will be slightly greater than that of the larger bubble. The pressure difference causes some movement of gas from the smaller bubble (decreasing its

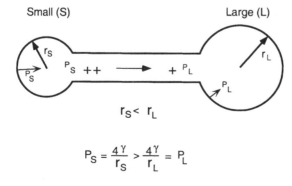

Figure 3.5. Schematic illustration showing two bubbles of different sizes connected through a tube. Because of the surface forces, pressure within the smaller bubble (P_S) exceeds that of the larger bubble (P_L). This leads to a flow of air from the smaller to the larger bubble and the eventual collapse of the smaller bubble.

radius and increasing its pressure) to the larger bubble (increasing its radius and decreasing its pressure). As a result, continuing movement causes a collapse of the smaller bubble with movement of gas into the larger bubble. The presence of surfactant in the alveolar liquid helps to prevent alveoli from coalescing because it reduces γ considerably.

Surfactant is synthesized within alveolar type II cells and is secreted into the alveolar lining liquid. Lamellar bodies of the type II cells provide storage sites for the lipoprotein. Surfactant is made up of many constituents, the major lipid being dipalmitoyl phosphatidylcholine (DPPC) and a protein that helps stabilize DPPC at the air–liquid interface.

Infant respiratory distress syndrome (IRDS), described in Chapter 12, is a disease with markedly reduced lung surfactant that can occur in premature infants. Reduced surfactant leads to increased alveolar surface forces. Atelectasis (alveolar collapse) and increased work of breathing are common with IRDS.

A remarkable feature of the surfactant in the liquid lining of the lung is its tendency to disrupt the intermolecular forces, and this decreases surface tension. This minimizes collapse of alveoli due to the liquid–air interface. The surface tension of lung surfactant changes with lung volume (Fig. 3.6). With expiration, the decreased surface area increases surfactant surface density, thereby decreasing surface tension. As the surface compresses, some surfactant is forced below the surface, forming small micelles (spherical surfactant globs). The opposite occurs with

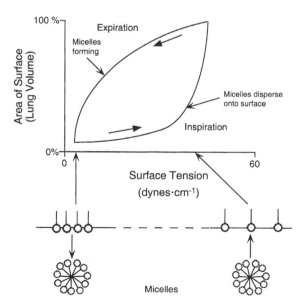

Figure 3.6. Relationship between surface tension and area of the surface film. During expiration, surfactant molecules on the surface move closer together, eventually causing some molecules to form micelles under the surface. During inspiration, surfactant molecules on the surface move further away, allowing surfactant molecules from the micelles to reenter the surface.

inspiration. Later during inspiration, the increased area available on the surface allows micelles to rise to the surface again and disperse an increasing number of surfactant molecules on the surface. The time required for micelle formation (expiration) and release (inspiration) causes some of the hysteresis (lack of superimposition of inspiration and expiration curves of air-filled lungs) shown in Figure 3.6. The current thinking is that most of the collapsed surfactant remains associated with the interface (surface-associated surfactant reservoir). Thus surfactant undergoes respreading instead of adsorption during expansion.

The importance of surface forces on the overall pressure–volume properties of the lung can be demonstrated by determining pressure–volume curves with saline and comparing these to pressure–volume curves with air. With saline inflation, the saline–air interface (and its contribution to work) is eliminated. Because the work for expanding the surface is not needed, saline inflation can be accomplished with less pressure (Fig. 3.7). There is no difference in the maximum lung volume, but there is a reduction in the relative hysteresis. Therefore, hysteresis of a normal lung pressure–volume relationship is due in part to the liquid–air surface, while some is also caused by inherent hysteresis of the stretching and relaxation of the lung parenchyma.

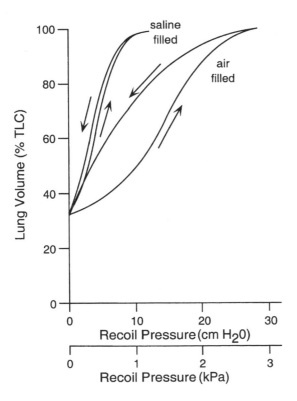

Figure 3.7. Pressure–volume curves for both air-filled and liquid-filled lungs. The presence of the air-liquid surface in air-filled lungs causes a greater difference in recoil pressures between inspiration and expiration, as well as increased hysteresis.

Interdependence in the Lung

Interdependence is a term referring to the influence of mechanical properties of alveoli on neighboring alveoli. The tendency toward alveolar collapse is also opposed by the tethering influence of lung parenchyma. This interdependence arises because the alveolar tissue is interconnected. If one alveolus begins to collapse, it stretches the collagen and elastin of the adjacent alveoli; this produces a force opposing further collapse. The lung parenchyma behaves like a large number of interconnected springs. Distortion of one spring leads to alteration in the nearby springs. Because the parenchyma is also connected to (intrapulmonary) airways, this interdependence also helps to maintain airway integrity and patency. The diameter of the intraparenchymal airways increases at larger lung volumes. To a certain extent, the interdependence also serves to make the ventilation distribution more uniform within the lung. With the development of diseases that break down lung tissue, such as emphysema, the role of this interdependence is reduced, and ventilation distribution becomes more heterogeneous (also referred to as *nonuniform* or *inhomogeneous*).

Dynamic Properties

Ventilation of gas into and out of the lungs is simply governed by the conversion of energy between two types: potential and kinetic. The *potential energy* of a gas is the stored energy, which equals the energy of each gas molecule multiplied by the number of molecules present. If gas density is increased due to a rise in pressure, a greater potential energy is stored within a given volume. *Kinetic energy* refers to the energy of gas molecules in bulk (convective) movement. More gas molecules moving in the same direction with higher velocity will have a higher kinetic energy. Gas moves from a region of higher potential energy, or pressure, to a region of lower pressure by flow, resulting in the conversion of potential energy to kinetic energy. Airflow, the movement of gas, is opposed by the frictional dissipation of kinetic energy due to the internal viscosity of gas as well as friction within the airway wall.

Pattern of Flow

Airflow within the airways can exist in two general patterns: laminar and turbulent (see Chapter 1). The laminar flow pattern is distorted when flow from two tubes converges into a single tube during exhalation or when flow separates and changes direction at a bifurcation during inhalation.

Whether gas flow is laminar or turbulent is determined by the flow rate and the geometry of the region. Airflow is normally laminar in smaller airways (small Reynolds number) and turbulent in larger airways (large Reynolds number), but the exact distribution depends on the breathing pattern.

Resistance

Air flow through the airway tree depends on the driving pressure and airway resistance:

$$\dot{V} = \frac{\Delta P}{R} = \frac{P_{atm} - P_A}{R} \qquad (3.7)$$

As discussed in Chapter 1, in any airway with laminar flow the resistance depends on geometric factors (length [ℓ] and radius [r] and gas viscosity (η):

$$R = \frac{8\eta\ell}{\pi r^4} \qquad (3.8)$$

Note the strong dependence of resistance on airway radius (to the fourth power).

A halving of radius results in a 16-fold increase in resistance. A significant change in airflow can result from very small changes in airway size. For the whole lung the airways' resistance reflects the complex combination of tubes of different sizes arranged both in parallel and in series. With progression into the distal airways, their number increases at a faster rate than the decrease in individual airway area. This results in a large increase in total airway cross-sectional area and, hence, a decrease in airflow velocity. Even though the individual airway radii are decreasing, the large increase in number of parallel airways and the decrease in flow rate results in a decrease in Reynolds number and a decrease in total airways' resistance with progression into the airway tree.

Maximal Flow

Increased inspiratory effort causes an increase in inspiratory flow. With increasing expiratory effort, however, collapse of very large airways limits the maximum achievable flow. A schematic representation of the flow limitation phenomenon is given in Figure 3.8. During inspiration, muscle contraction causes a negative alveolar pressure and, at any location in the airways, a negative intraairway pressure. Because pleural pressure is always lower than alveolar pressure (due to static lung recoil), the pleural pressure is always more negative than intraairway pressure,

Inspiration

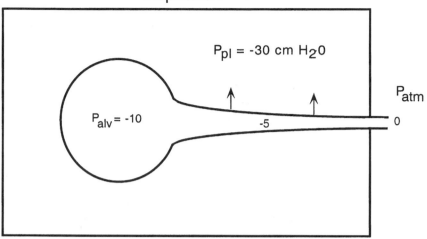

Rapid Expiration

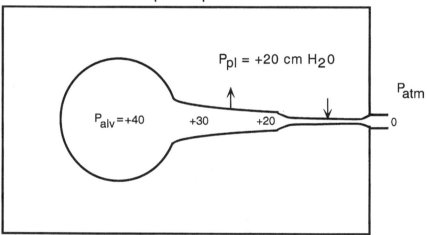

Figure 3.8. Schematic illustration of airway and pleural pressures during inspiration **(top)** and dynamic compression of rapid expiration **(bottom)**. During forced expiration, upper airways collapse when the pleural pressure exceeds intraairway pressure. (Adapted from B. Culver, Ed., Human Biology 541 syllabus: *The Respiratory System.* University of Washington, Seattle: ASUW Publishing.)

resulting in a net distending force on the walls of the extraparenchymal, intrathoracic airways, which keeps them open.

The strong effort of a rapid exhalation causes a positive pleural pressure. Because of lung recoil, alveolar pressure will exceed pleural pressure. As airflow proceeds along the airways, pressure decreases due to energy loss caused by the airway resistance. Eventually the intraairway pressure will be less than the pleural pressure, resulting in an inward force and collapse of the airways. In addition, Bernoulli effects* accentuate this compression because the total cross-sectional area of the airways falls to a minimum in collapsed airways, and gas velocities must therefore be highest at this location. This phenomenon occurs in airways that are outside the lung parenchyma (and not subject to its tethering effect) but within the thorax (and subject to the compressive effect of the positive extraairway, pleural pressure). These airways have a C-shaped cartilage connected by a distensible membrane that invaginates into the airway lumen during forced exhalation because of the inwardly directed pressure difference. The marked decrease in airway cross-sectional area produces a large increase in the linear velocity of flow, a mechanism that helps to clear the airways during a cough.

Flow–Volume Curve

The flow–volume curve shown in Figure 3.9 illustrates a common means of analyzing the flow properties of the respiratory system. Exhaled flow is plotted against lung volume. With a small amount of expiratory effort, flow increases to a relatively low value and remains constant at that value while lung volume decreases. Eventually, as lung volume approaches RV, airway resistance increases and respiratory muscle pressure decreases so that flow declines toward zero at RV. With an intermediate effort, expiratory flow is greater until the maximal flow curve is reached. When this occurs the flow declines linearly with lung volume, approaching zero flow at RV. With maximal effort, flow rises rapidly to a peak as maximal flow is achieved and then declines to zero flow at RV. At high lung volume, airways are large and the flow is effort dependent; greater effort results in greater flow. At lower lung volume, airways are smaller and airway flow is independent of effort. Beyond a certain minimum alveolar pressure, flow is effort independent; greater effort causes a proportionally greater airway resistance while flow remains constant.

At higher lung volumes during expiration, the parenchymal tethering of airways makes the resistance of the smaller airways very low. At lower lung volumes, the relative contribution of small airway resistance becomes greater as the size of

---

*Bernoulli noted that the sum of kinetic and potential energy must remain constant. When airflow enters a constriction, linear velocity increases, and therefore pressure must decrease. This decrease in pressure promotes airway collapse.

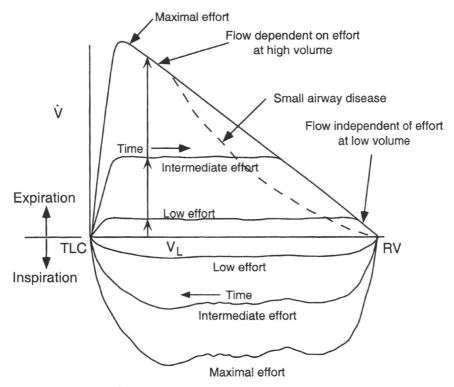

Figure 3.9. Representative flow–volume curves in a normal subject for three levels of effort. Expiratory and inspiratory curves are shown.

these airways diminishes. When patients with airway disease develop thickened bronchial mucosa, small airway resistance increases and becomes more important at lower lung volumes during exhalation. This gives curvilinearity to the flow-independent portion of the flow–volume curve (see Fig. 3.9), a property that is sometimes used to help diagnose small airway disease.

During inspiration, the flow is proportional to effort. No flow limitation is seen because the airways are expanded due to the negative pleural pressure.

Isovolume Pressure–Flow Curve

The data from flow–volume curves, plotted on isovolume pressure–flow curves (Fig. 3.10), reveal some information about the lungs. Flow is plotted against alveolar pressure for a specific lung volume from different flow–volume curves (Fig. 3.9). Each curve crosses the horizontal (zero-flow) axis at zero alveolar pressure.

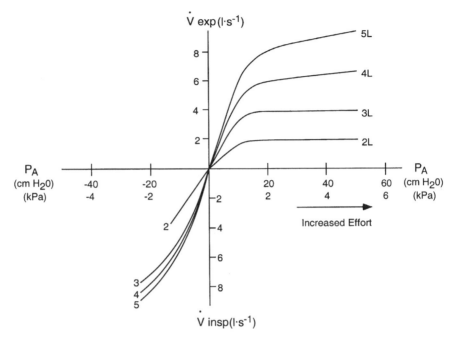

Figure 3.10. Isovolume pressure–flow curves. The data from Figure 3.9 are replotted to show flow versus alveolar pressure. Data points are taken from flow–volume curves performed with different levels of effort.

The slope of the curve at zero flow is the inverse of airway resistance ($\dot{V}/\Delta P$). With decreasing alveolar pressure, inspiratory flow occurs, and this flow is proportional to the difference between alveolar pressure and atmospheric pressure. The greater role of turbulent flow at higher flow rates causes a nonlinearity in the inspiratory portion of the isovolume pressure–flow curve. As alveolar pressure increases from the zero flow point, expiratory flow increases. As alveolar pressure becomes increasingly positive, flow eventually achieves a maximum that is dependent on lung volume. Figure 3.10 also shows that, at lower lung volumes, the maximum expiration flow rate is independent of effort (increasing alveolar pressure).

Obstructive Lung Disease

The normal mechanical function of the lung is disturbed in the presence of obstructive lung disease, a general class of disease that results in increased airway resistance. Obstructive diseases fall into three general types: chronic bronchitis, asthma, and emphysema. In chronic bronchitis, airway resistance rises because of a decrease in airway diameter due to increased mucus production. Asthma causes a narrowing of the airways due to an increase in tone of airway smooth muscle, usually in response to an antigen. Emphysema causes a loss (destruction) of parenchyma that decreases the airway tethering and increases airway resistance.

The normal mechanical function of the lung is altered in obstructive lung disease (Fig. 3.11). The increased airway resistance leads to a reduced volume that can be exhaled in a certain period of time. A normal individual exhales around 75% to 80% of vital capacity per second (FEV_1/VC). This is reduced to lower fractions of vital capacity as the degree of obstructive disease increases. To breathe easier (less work), a patient with obstructive disease typically breathes at larger lung volumes (increasing airway diameter) and has a larger RV because the airways close sooner during exhalation. Finally, patients with long-term obstructive disease may increase TLC as stronger inspiratory muscles are developed.

Restrictive Lung Disease

Volume-reducing diseases are called *restrictive lung diseases*. Typical restrictive diseases include fibrosis, silicosis, asbestosis, scoliosis and volume-occupying tumors. Spirometry of a typical patient with restrictive disease shows reduction in all lung volumes, including a marked reduction in VC and TLC (Fig. 3.11). There is a normal, or possibly increased, FEV_1/VC. These patients usually demonstrate a decreased compliance of the total respiratory system.

Work of Breathing

The amount of energy or work required for breathing has two components: (*1*) the work of stretching the lung and chest wall (elastic work) and (*2*) the energy dissipated by the convective movement of air through the airways (resistive work). Most of the elastic energy of inspiration is stored in the stretched fibers, which then provide the energy needed for exhalation. Work can be estimated from the pressure–volume relationship (Fig. 3.12) by integrating pressure with respect to volume over the entire respiratory cycle:

$$W = \int PdV \qquad (3.9)$$

The hatched areas in Figure 3.12 indicate the work for normal inspiratory and expiratory effort. The amount of work for each curve is represented by the area between the curve and the vertical axis. The work of inspiration includes an elastic

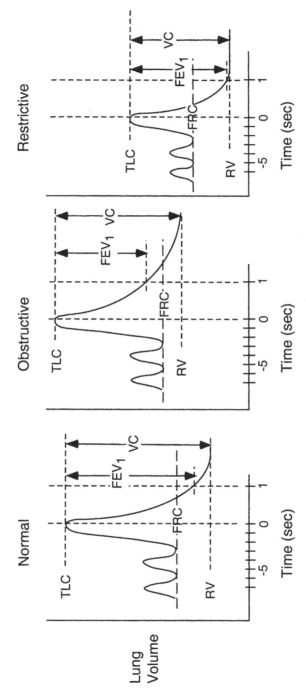

Figure 3.11. Spirometry curves for normal subjects and patients with either obstructive or restrictive disease. Lung volume is plotted against time. The time scale changes at time 0 when the subject exhales as rapidly as possible. Flow is the slope of the line at any point. Note that lung volumes are generally increased and flows are decreased in obstructive disease. In restrictive diseases, lung volumes are decreased while flows remain relatively normal.

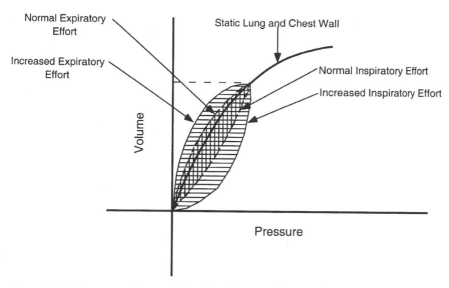

Figure 3.12. Pressure–volume relationships in normal lungs with normal and increased effort. Cross-hatched shading represents the work of breathing for a normal inspiration and expiration. Horizontal line shading shows the work of breathing for both inspiration and expiration for increased effort.

component (area between the static curve and the vertical axis) and a dynamic component (area between the static curve and the actual curve). The difference between the two is the resistive work of one breath. The wider flaring of the increased effort curves shows much greater resistive work.

The total work of breathing is the sum of elastic and resistive work. Figure 3.13 is a schematic representation of how total work of breathing changes with changing lung volume. Total work is the sum of resistive work, which decreases with increasing lung volume and widening airways, and elastic work, which increases at both high and low lung volumes. Total work for normal lungs is minimal at an end-exhaled lung volume near FRC.

In obstructive lung disease, resistive work increases with no change in elastic work. The result is an increase in total work at any lung volume. The patient breathes at a higher FRC to reduce the resistive and, hence, total work of breathing.

In restrictive lung disease, elastic work increases with no change in resistive work. The result is, again, an increase in total work at any lung volume. The patient breathes at a lower FRC to reduce the elastic and, hence, total work of breathing. The cost of a lower FRC is an increase in the resistive work of breathing.

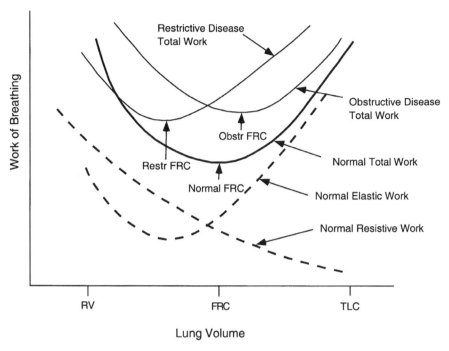

Figure 3.13. Work of breathing is shown for normal subjects and patients with obstructive or restrictive disease. Dashed lines show the elastic and resistive work for a normal subject. In obstructive disease, the resistive work increases. In restrictive disease, the elastic work increases.

Under normal circumstances, the amount of energy required for breathing amounts to 1% to 2% of total body oxygen consumption at rest. The relative work of breathing can, however, increase substantially in severe exercise.

Intubation and Mechanical Ventilation

For critically ill patients when there is a need to bypass the upper airway or in situations of respiratory failure and mechanical ventilation is warranted, intubation is required. The most common form of intubation is endotracheal intubation and involves passing a tube first through the mouth and then through the larynx so that the end of the tube lies in the trachea below the level of the larynx. When this cannot be accomplished or is undesirable, a tracheostomy is performed. This involves making an incision in the skin overlying the trachea and then opening the anterior wall of the trachea between a pair of cartilaginous tracheal rings; the subject can then breathe or be mechanically ventilated through this opening.

Patients often require assistance with breathing in order to minimize the work of breathing. With a mechanical ventilator, air is delivered to the patient; positive pressure is used to expand the lung and inflate the lungs either to a given tidal volume (volume ventilation) or a given end-inspired pressure (pressure ventilation). Exhalation is caused by opening the exhalation valve and allowing the increased alveolar pressure to result in passive exhalation.

Increasing lung volume during mechanical ventilation can improve gas exchange efficiency. This can be accomplished by application of positive end-expiratory pressure (PEEP), which requires that the patient exhale against a pressure that will maintain an increased lung volume at end exhalation. The increased lung volume with PEEP helps to maintain a larger lung volume and minimize small airway collapse at the end of exhalation. A potential problem at higher PEEP levels is the risk of reducing cardiac output due to the higher alveolar pressures through-out the respiratory cycle.

Distribution of Ventilation

Ventilation does not distribute uniformly to all alveoli. In part, convective factors govern ventilation distribution. The relative efficiency of mixing inspired gas with the gas initially in the alveoli is, however, thought to depend on a combination of convection-related and diffusion-related mechanisms.

The classic framework with which to analyze ventilation develops from a gravity-dependent distribution model (Fig. 3.14). Because the lungs are suspended within the thorax in the erect human, the pull of gravity causes a greater distention of the upper lung than of the lower lung due to the greater weight of the lung pulling down on the upper alveoli. This results in a pleural pressure that is more negative at the top than at the bottom. The upper lung alveoli are thus higher on their pressure–volume curve. With inspiration, the pleural pressure is increased equally in all regions of the lung. Because the lower lung has a greater effective compliance, it will receive more ventilation than the top. Although the vertical distribution of compliance plays a major role in the distribution of ventilation, recent studies with high-resolution methods have identified a component of venti-lation distribution determined by airway resistance variation.

With exhalation below FRC toward RV, the lower part of the lung may reach a positive pleural pressure, resulting in closure of the airways. Stopping airflow to those alveoli distal to a closed airway reduces their ventilation. This so-called clos-ing volume (lung volume at which airway closure begins) increases with lung

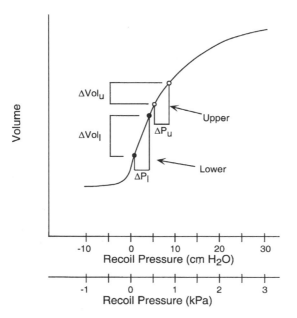

Figure 3.14. Schematic illustration demonstrating nonuniformity of the lung during normal ventilation. Both the upper (u) and lower (l) portions of the lungs fall on the same pressure–volume curve. Recoil pressure in the lower lung is less than that in the upper lung. The same change in pressure results in greater ventilation to the lower lung with the greater compliance.

disease (particularly obstructive) and with age in normal individuals. If the closing volume exceeds FRC, some alveoli will receive no ventilation during part of the ventilatory cycle.

When patients with lung disease are changed from the supine (face upward) to the prone (face downward) position, the normal vertical gradient in pleural pressure observed in the erect and supine positions disappears, causing a more uniform ventilation distribution. Rotating patients to the prone position has been shown to improve gas exchange in a majority of patients with adult respiratory disease syndrome (a pulmonary edema resulting from inflammation or trauma) as well as those with pulmonary edema.

It is clear, however, that the distribution of ventilation is not determined solely by gravity. During inspiration, the expanding parenchyma is distorted by the relatively rigid large airways, resulting in local differences in airway resistance. An additional factor affecting the uniformity of ventilation is the shape of the lung. When outside the chest, the lung takes on a shape different from the inner surface of the chest wall. Therefore, *in vivo*, the lung is distorted from its natural shape. During inspiration, the expansion of the chest wall and lung is not identical at each position along the surface of the lungs because the mechanics of rib expansion is different from the mechanics of lung parenchyma expansion. This irregularity causes some additional heterogeneity of ventilation.

Further Reading

1. Altose, M D. Pulmonary Mechanics. In: *Fishman A P, editor. Pulmonary Diseases and Disorders*, vol 1. New York: McGraw-Hill, 1998, pp 149–162.
2. Hoppin F G, Stothert J C Jr, Greaves I A, Lai Y L, Hildebrandt J. Lung recoil: Elastic and rheological properties. In: Farhi L E, Tenney S M, editors. *Handbook of Physiology*, Section 3, *The Respiratory System*, vol III, *Mechanics of Breathing*, part 1. Bethesda, MD: American Physiological Society, 1986, pp 195–215.
3. Hughes J M B, N B Pride. *Lung Function Tests: Physiological Principles and Clinical Applications*. London: W B. Saunders, 1999.
4. Levitsky, M G. *Pulmonary Physiology*, (5th ed.) New York: McGraw-Hill, 1999.
5. Lumb A B. *Nunn's Applied Respiratory Physiology*, (5th ed.) Oxford: Butterworth-Heinemann, 2000.
6. Schürch S, Bachofen H, Possmeyer F. Alveolar lining layer. Functions, composition, structures. In: Hlastala M P, Robertson H T, editors. *Lung Biology in Health and Disease*, vol. 121, *Complexity in Structure and Function of the Lung*. New York: Marcel Dekker, 1998, pp 35–98.

Study Questions

3.1. Use pressure–volume curves of the lung, chest wall, and respiratory system to explain the changes in elastic properties of the respiratory system in restrictive disease caused by a space-occupying lesion.

3.2. How deep can a person go under water while breathing from above the surface through a tube? Consider problems with resistance and maximal respiratory muscle effort.

3.3. Hyaline membrane disease is an abnormality of premature newborns with insufficient surfactant in their lungs. What is the effect on stability of alveoli in the lungs?

3.4. Explain how expired flow is limited during maximal expiration, but not during relaxed expiration.

3.5. What are the expected changes in the lung volumes and airway resistance with obstructive disease and changes in lung volumes with restrictive disease?

3.6. A patient requiring positive pressure ventilation (air forced into the lungs by a ventilator with pressure) is given a tidal volume of 0.8 l. The pressure dial on the ventilator rises to 30 cm H_2O with each breath but falls to 24 cm H_2O at the end of inspiration (best seen if the lungs are briefly held at the end-inspiratory volume by transiently occluding expiration). During expiration the pressure at the airway opening is zero. Calculate the compliance observed over this tidal inflation. Is this the compliance of lung, chest wall, or both? If the recoil pressure of this patient's lungs is 25 cm H_2O at the end-inspiratory volume, what is the intrapleural pressure at this time?

3.7. A patient inhales by mouth at a rate of 0.5 l · sec^{-1}. At the instant his lung volume is 3.0 l, the pleural pressure (measured via an esophageal balloon) is -7 cm H_2O. His static lung recoil at 3.0 l is 5 cm H_2O. Calculate airway resistance (R_{aw}) and discuss this in relation to normal values. What would you expect his esophageal pressure to be at the same lung volume when he exhales at 0.4 l · sec^{-1}?

4

Ventilation

Efficient transfer of gases in the lung requires that blood and inspired air be brought into close proximity. Ventilation is described as the movement of fresh air from outside the body to the alveoli, where gas exchange occurs, and the subsequent movement of alveolar gas back to the outside.

Inspired Air

Outside air consists of gases (see Chapter 1) in a ratio of approximately 21% O_2 and 79% nitrogen with varying water vapor, depending on temperature and humidity, that dilutes the gases accordingly. How to deal with dry gas mixtures using fractions and partial pressures and taking into account the influence of water vapor is covered in Chapter 1.

With inspiration, outside air is heated to body temperature and humidified by evaporation from the airway mucosa. After air reaches the more distal airways completely heated (37°C) and humidified (100% saturated at 37°C), the inspired partial pressure of O_2 (PI_{O_2}) can be calculated as

$$PI_{O_2} = FI_{O_2} (P_B - P_{H_2O}) \tag{4.1}$$
$$= 0.21 (760 - 47) = 0.21 \times 713 = 150 \text{ mm Hg}$$
$$PI_{N_2} = 0.79 \times 713 = 563 \text{ mm Hg}$$

Total Ventilation

The total ventilation, or minute volume, can be determined by collecting exhaled gas for a measured time ($\dot{V}_E$ = volume exhaled per minute). The volume of gas exhaled during one normal respiratory cycle is known as the tidal volume (V_T). Total ventilation is equal to the average tidal volume multiplied by the breathing frequency (f):

$$\dot{V}_E = V_T \cdot f \qquad (4.2)$$

Alveolar Ventilation

Gas exchange occurs in the alveolar acinus when fresh air comes in close proximity to capillary blood. Not all inspired air, however, reaches the alveoli to participate in gas exchange (Fig. 4.1). The inspired air must first pass through the conducting airways: the nose, mouth, pharynx, larynx, trachea, bronchi, and bronchioles. These airways conduct air from the atmosphere to the alveoli. Because airways contain no alveoli (at least up to the terminal bronchioles; see Chapter 2), they do not participate in respiratory gas exchange. They do, however, participate in the warming and humidification of inspired air. At the end of inspiration, the volume of inspired air remaining in the conducting airways is known as the *anatomical dead space* ("dead" because it does not participate in O_2 and CO_2 exchange). The effect of the conducting airways on ventilation and gas exchange can be considered in two ways. After inspiration, humidified and warmed atmospheric air remains in these airways and is the first gas exhaled on the subsequent exhalation. After expiration, alveolar gas (with CO_2 added and O_2 partially removed) fills the anatomical dead space and reenters the alveoli with the next breath. Thus a tidal breath may consist of 600 ml of inspired air that will cause a 600 ml expansion of the alveolar volume followed by exhalation of 600 ml. The volume of fresh air deliv-

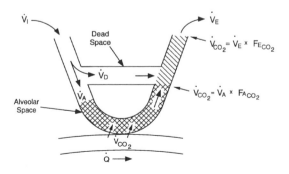

Figure 4.1. Schematic diagram of ventilation in the lung. Inspired ventilation is divided between the dead space and the alveolar space, where it picks up CO_2. Upon exhalation, ventilation from the dead space ($\dot{V}_D$) and from the alveolar space ($\dot{V}_A$) combine to form the total ventilation ($\dot{V}_E$). The lung is perfused by pulmonary blood flow ($\dot{Q}$).

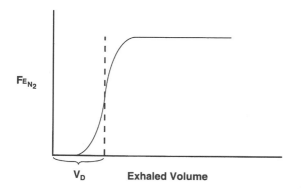

V_D **Exhaled Volume**

Figure 4.2. Measurement of anatomical dead space (V_D). After a single inspiration of 100% O_2, exhaled nitrogen concentration (FE_{N_2}) is measured as a function of exhaled volume. Anatomical dead space is the exhaled volume to the point of transition between dead space and alveolar gas.

ered to the alveoli and the volume of alveolar air exhaled to the atmosphere will each be less than 600 ml by the volume of the anatomical dead space.

The anatomical dead space can be measured after an inspiration of 100% O_2. Figure 4.2 shows the expired partial pressure profile of N_2 versus expired volume. The initial exhalate consists of air from the anatomical dead space, which has no N_2 after O_2 inspiration. Exhaled alveolar air has N_2. Drawing a vertical line through the midpoint of the transition phase allows calculation of the anatomical dead space volume.

In addition to the conducting airways, any alveoli that are ventilated with air, but not perfused with blood, do not participate in gas exchange. The volume of ventilation going to these alveoli also acts as dead space ventilation and is known as *alveolar dead space*. Ventilation to areas of lung with reduced perfusion behaves as if a portion were going to alveoli with normal perfusion and a portion to alveoli with no perfusion. This latter portion is also part of the alveolar dead space, as shown schematically in Figure 4.3. The sum of anatomical and alveolar dead spaces makes up the physiological dead space.

$$V_{D_{physiol}} = V_{D_{anat}} + V_{D_{alv}} \qquad (4.3)$$

In this chapter, the abbreviations V_D and $\dot{V}_D$ without further qualifiers refer to the physiological dead space and its ventilation, respectively. The physiological dead space (V_D), or wasted ventilation ($\dot{V}_D$), is usually expressed as a fraction of the tidal volume (V_D/V_T) or of total ventilation ($\dot{V}_D/\dot{V}_E$).

The physiological dead space may increase with lung disease due primarily to an increased $\dot{V}_A/\dot{Q}$ heterogeneity and the alveolar dead space component (see Chapter 7). The volume of air that participates in gas exchange, because it is in contact with perfused alveoli, is known as *alveolar ventilation* ($\dot{V}_A = \dot{V}_E - \dot{V}_{D_{physiol}}$). The volume per minute of alveolar ventilation is critical, as it determines

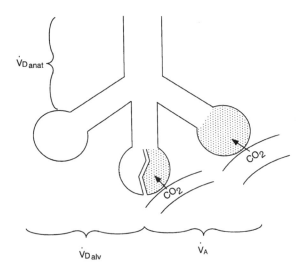

Figure 4.3. Schematic illustration of dead space ventilation. Physiological dead space (V_D) is composed of anatomical dead space ($V_{D_{anat}}$) plus alveolar dead space ($V_{D_{alv}}$). (Adapted from B. Culver, Ed., Human Biology 541 syllabus: *The Respiratory System*. University of Washington, Seattle. ASUW Publishing.)

the amount of air presented to alveoli into which CO_2 can be added and from which O_2 can be removed.

Alveolar Gas Composition

Carbon Dioxide Exchange

CO_2 production is eliminated from the body only by ventilation. $\dot{V}_{CO_2}$ equals the volume of CO_2 exhaled per minute ($\dot{V}E_{CO_2}$) minus the volume of CO_2 inhaled (negligible). Because CO_2 in the expired gas must have come from alveolar ventilation (Fig. 4.1),

$$\dot{V}_{CO_2} = \dot{V}_A \, FA_{CO_2} = \dot{V}_E \, FE_{CO_2} \tag{4.4}$$

where FA_{CO_2} is the concentration of CO_2 in the alveolar space and FE_{CO_2} is the concentration of CO_2 in mixed expired gas. From this equation, a relationship between PA_{CO_2} and ventilation can be derived (see appendix at the end of this chapter).

$$PA_{CO_2} = \frac{\dot{V}_{CO_2}}{\dot{V}_A} (P_B - 47) \tag{4.5}$$

This relationship, called the *alveolar ventilation equation* is very important. Alveolar P_{CO_2} is directly related to the metabolic production of CO_2 and inversely related to alveolar ventilation. The body maintains a normal arterial and alveolar P_{CO_2} of 40 ± 3 mm Hg by adjusting ventilation appropriately for the $\dot{V}_{CO_2}$ determined by metabolism. When equation 4.5 is used, both $\dot{V}_A$ and $\dot{V}_{CO_2}$ must be expressed in the same units and under the same conditions (i.e., either body temperature, ambient pressure, saturated [BTPS] or standard temperature and pressure, dry [STPD]). This is particularly important when the individual is at high altitude.

Hyperventilation is defined as ventilation in excess of metabolic needs. It follows from the alveolar ventilation equation that PA_{CO_2} less than normal (<37 mm Hg) indicates alveolar hyperventilation. Conversely, a PA_{CO_2} greater than normal (>43 mm Hg) indicates alveolar hypoventilation. Alveolar ventilation can be altered by changes in either total ventilation or wasted ventilation ($\dot{V}_A = \dot{V}_E - \dot{V}_D$). Any depression in central nervous system function can alter $\dot{V}_E$; for example, many drugs such as analgesics and sedatives can reduce $\dot{V}_E$. Any increase in $\dot{V}_D$ will reduce $\dot{V}_A$ unless $\dot{V}_E$ increases accordingly. Many disease processes increase physiological dead space and PA_{CO_2}. In severe obstructive lung disease, CO_2 retention may lead to respiratory failure when the patient can no longer increase total ventilation because of the high work of breathing.

PA_{CO_2} reflects a balance between CO_2 delivery to the alveoli ($\dot{V}A_{CO_2}$) and CO_2 elimination from the lungs by ventilation ($\dot{V}A_{CO_2}$). In a steady state, production and excretion must be the same. Under resting conditions $\dot{V}_{CO_2}$ is relatively constant at approximately 200 ml(STPD) · min^{-1} for a normal-sized individual at rest. With transient hyperventilation CO_2 will be exhaled at a greater rate than it is produced; PA_{CO_2} (and arterial [a] P_{CO_2}) will fall. As PA_{CO_2} falls, the CO_2 exhaled per minute will decrease until it is again equal to CO_2 production and a new steady state is established. With hypoventilation, the rate of CO_2 exhalation falls initially; then PA_{CO_2} (and Pa_{CO_2}) rises until a new steady state is reached where excretion again equals production, but now with less ventilation and with each liter of gas leaving the alveoli carrying more CO_2. This mechanism allows patients with severe lung disease and high work of breathing to excrete their CO_2 production at less energy cost due to hypoventilation and higher PA_{CO_2}.

The principles in equation 4.4 are often used to measure $\dot{V}_{CO_2}$. The clinical "open-circuit" technique requires all expired gas from an individual to be collected in a bag for a fixed period of time (e.g., 1 minute). After one measures the volume of gas in the bag and the CO_2 fraction of that gas, the $\dot{V}_{CO_2}$ can be calculated. Similarly, $\dot{V}_{O_2}$ can be determined from a measurement of FE_{O_2}, FI_{O_2}, and $\dot{V}_E$.

Respiratory Quotient

Energy necessary for life processes arises from the oxidation of carbohydrates, protein, and fats, producing mainly CO_2 and H_2O as breakdown products. The respiratory quotient (RQ) is the ratio of metabolic CO_2 production to the O_2 consumption ($\dot{V}_{CO_2}/\dot{V}_{O_2}$) of the tissues. When carbohydrate is metabolized, the RQ = 1.0:

$$C_6H_{12}O_6 + 6\ O_2 = 6\ CO_2 + 6\ H_2O \qquad (4.6)$$

$$RQ = \frac{\dot{V}_{CO_2}}{\dot{V}_{O_2}} = \frac{6}{6} = 1 \qquad (4.7)$$

When fat is metabolized, RQ is approximately 0.7. The RQ of protein metabolism is about 0.8. Thus the RQ for the entire body varies with the percentages of carbohydrate, fat, and protein being oxidized at any given time. The respiratory exchange ratio (R) relates the volume of CO_2 eliminated by the lungs to the net volume of O_2 taken up from the lungs. In a steady state or over a long period of time, R must equal RQ, but R may vary transiently with factors other than metabolism. If an individual suddenly increases ventilation, R rises because CO_2 is being blown off from blood and tissue stores. In contrast, this maneuver will not increase $\dot{V}_{O_2}$ to a similar degree, largely due to the relative flatness of the O_2 equilibrium curve and the low effective solubility of O_2 (Chapter 6).

Oxygen Exchange

The level of alveolar O_2 also reflects a balance of two processes: O_2 delivery to the alveoli by ventilation and O_2 removal from the alveoli by capillary blood and O_2 removal by exhaled air. Oxygen delivery to alveoli is determined by the ventilation ($\dot{V}_A$) and the fraction of inspired O_2 (FI_{O_2}). The air leaving alveoli has an alveolar O_2 concentration (FA_{O_2}); the net O_2 delivery is determined by $\dot{V}_A$ (FI_{O_2} − FA_{O_2}). Oxygen removal from the alveoli is governed by tissue O_2 consumption. Tissue $\dot{V}_{O_2}$ varies with disease and activity, but under resting conditions it is approximately 250 ml(STPD) · min^{-1} for an average-sized person. Under constant conditions, the alveolar O_2 level is unchanged, so these processes of delivery and removal are equal. Thus the relationship between PA_{O_2} and $\dot{V}_{O_2}$ can be written as a parallel relationship to the alveolar ventilation equation (see appendix at the end of this chapter):

$$PI_{O_2} - PA_{O_2} = \frac{\dot{V}_{O_2}}{\dot{V}_A} (P_B - 47) \qquad (4.8)$$

Equation 4.8 is analogous to the alveolar ventilation equation (Eq. 4.5) for CO_2. It shows that PA_{O_2} is determined only by PI_{O_2}, $\dot{V}_A$, and $\dot{V}_{O_2}$. If PI_{O_2} and $\dot{V}_{O_2}$ remain constant and $\dot{V}_A$ rises (hyperventilation), then PA_{O_2} must increase, and, if $\dot{V}_A$ decreases (hypoventilation), then PA_{O_2} must also decrease.

Because $\dot{V}_{O_2}$ refers to the metabolic product of O_2 consumption, the quantities $\dot{V}_{CO_2}$ and $\dot{V}_{O_2}$ are linked to one another. If they are identical ($R = 1$), then the right sides of equations 4.5 and 4.8 are identical and show that the fall in P_{O_2} from inspired to alveolar air to be the same as the rise in P_{CO_2} from 0 to the alveolar level.

$$P_{A_{O_2}} = P_{I_{O_2}} - \frac{P_{A_{CO_2}}}{R} \qquad (4.9)$$

This well-known relationship, termed the *alveolar gas equation*, is often used to calculate the alveolar P_{O_2}.

When R is less than 1, more O_2 is removed from than CO_2 is added to the alveolar gas. For typical normal values [$R = 0.8$; $P_{I_{O_2}} = 0.21 (760 - 47)$ mm Hg; $P_{A_{CO_2}} = 40$ mm Hg]:

$$P_{A_{O_2}} = 150 \text{ mm Hg} - \frac{40 \text{ mm Hg}}{0.8} = 100 \text{ mm Hg} \qquad (4.10)$$

Equation 4.9 is frequently misinterpreted as indicating that alveolar O_2 is displaced by CO_2. This is incorrect, as the removal of O_2 and the addition of CO_2 proceed as independent processes in the lung. If the normal RQ in the tissues is assumed to be equal to 1, then the loss of O_2 from the inspired air to the blood is approximately equal to the gain in CO_2.

The most complete form of the alveolar gas equation accounts for the different diluting effect of inert gas (predominantly N_2) with changes in $F_{I_{O_2}}$:

$$P_{A_{O_2}} = P_{I_{O_2}} - P_{a_{O_2}} \left[F_{I_{O_2}} + \frac{(1 - F_{I_{O_2}})}{R} \right] \qquad (4.11)$$

The use of equation 4.11 is more accurate, but a bit more cumbersome, than equation 4.9. When the values in equation 4.10 are used, for example, the $P_{A_{O_2}}$ calculated with equation 4.11 is 102.1 mm Hg instead of 100 mm Hg. This simplification results in an error of only 2%. For a person breathing 100% oxygen ($F_{I_{O_2}} = 1$), equation 4.11 shows that the sum of $P_{a_{CO_2}}$ and $P_{A_{O_2}}$ always equals $P_{I_{O_2}}$ for any R.

The effect of changes in ventilation on alveolar O_2 and CO_2 is shown in Figure 4.4. Hyperventilation, an increase in ventilation relative to the metabolic CO_2 production, decreases P_{CO_2} and increases P_{O_2}. On the other hand, hypoventilation results in alveolar hypercapnia and hypoxia. Note that hypoventilation can dramatically affect $P_{A_{O_2}}$, particularly for lower R values.

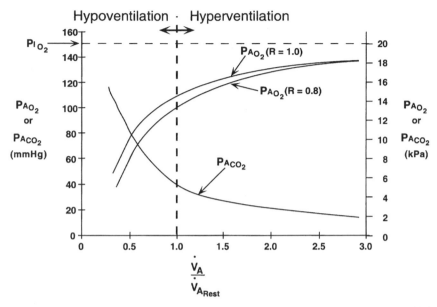

Figure 4.4. Changes in alveolar gases caused by changes in ventilation. Hyperventilation lowers PA_{CO_2} and raises PA_{O_2}. Hypoventilation raises PA_{CO_2} and lowers PA_{O_2}.

Nitrogen Exchange

When R is not equal to 1, $\dot{V}_{CO_2}$ is not equal to $\dot{V}_{O_2}$. Under such circumstances, the total amount of gas in the alveolus is altered as gas exchange occurs. Because the solubility of N_2 is very low, the total number of N_2 molecules in the alveolus remains unchanged. If the alveolar gas volume decreases (when $R < 1$), the relative fractions of N_2 and P_{N_2} increase. On the other hand, when $R > 1$, alveolar gas volume increases, the relative fractions of N_2 and P_{N_2} decrease. Under usual circumstances, if the overall R is about 0.8, the alveolar P_{N_2} (and alveolar endcapillary blood P_{N_2}) is about 10 mm Hg greater than inspired P_{N_2} (humidified). Expired P_{N_2} exceeds inspired P_{N_2} even though there is essentially no net nitrogen exchange.

Both alveolar P_{O_2} and P_{CO_2} change during the respiratory cycle because ventilation is periodic, while $\dot{V}_{O_2}$ and $\dot{V}_{CO_2}$ are relatively constant. During inspiration, fresh air is delivered to the alveolus, causing P_{CO_2} to decrease and P_{O_2} to increase (Fig. 4.5). During expiration, continued gas exchange causes P_{CO_2} to increase and P_{O_2} to decrease. Even though the alveolar gas equations predict constant values for P_{CO_2} and P_{O_2}, the values actually fluctuate about the mean values by ± 0.7 mm Hg and ± 2.2 mm Hg for P_{CO_2} and P_{CO_2}, respectively.

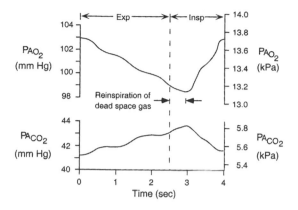

Figure 4.5. Alveolar P_{O_2} and P_{CO_2} fluctuations during a single respiratory cycle. The large oscillation is caused by periodic ventilation. Small oscillations are caused by pulsatile pulmonary blood flow. (Adapted from Hlastala MP. A model of fluctuating alveolar gas exchange during the respiratory cycle. *Respir Physiol* 15:214–232, 1972, with permission.)

Dead Space Ventilation

Anatomical Dead Space

The volume of the anatomical dead space in a normal adult male is 150 to 180 ml (a commonly used approximation is that the V_D in ml equals lean body weight in lb). In a young, normal individual, the volume of the physiological dead space is only slightly greater, about 25% to 35% of an average tidal volume (referred to as the V_D/V_T ratio). The V_D/V_T ratio does not remain constant under all conditions. Changes in ventilation can result from changes in either tidal volume or respiratory frequency (Fig. 4.6). Increasing frequency while maintaining constant tidal volume will result in the same fraction of tidal volume going to both dead space and alveolar space increasing $\dot{V}_D$ and $\dot{V}_A$ in proportion to the increase in $\dot{V}_E$, with no change in V_D/V_T. Increasing tidal volume while maintaining a constant frequency will result in no change in $\dot{V}_D$ and an increase in $\dot{V}_A$. The result is a progressive decrease in V_D/V_T.

The anatomical dead space is not fixed but increases at higher lung volumes because the intrapulmonary airways increase in size along with the surrounding lung tissue. Thus, breathing with an increased tidal volume and increased end-inspiratory lung volume is associated with a smaller decrease in V_D/V_T ratio than that shown in Figure 4.6.

With exercise, tidal volume may increase to 2.5 to 3.0 l and V_D/V_T normally falls to 10% to 15% (see Chapter 12). This is caused in part by an increase in pulmonary blood flow, which tends to eliminate any poorly perfused alveolar dead space. At the other extreme, it would seem that as tidal volume became small and approached the anatomical dead space, alveolar ventilation would fall to zero and

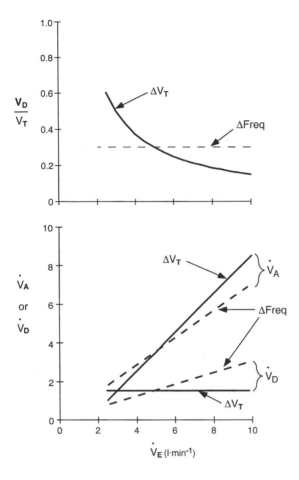

Figure 4.6. Changes in dead space ventilation and alveolar ventilation **(lower)** and anatomical dead space to tidal volume ratio **(upper)** with changes in overall ventilation. Dashed curves show changes when breathing frequency is varied at a constant tidal volume. Solid curves indicate changes when tidal volume is varied at a constant frequency, causing a change in the relative amount of the tidal volume going to dead space versus the alveolar region.

gas exchange would be impossible. It has, however, been demonstrated that gas exchange can be maintained even with tidal volumes equal to or smaller than the measured anatomical dead space if ventilation occurs at a high enough frequency. Some fresh gas reaches alveoli because of physical mixing induced by high breathing frequencies.

Physiological Dead Space

The ventilation wasted by ventilating dead space includes that going to anatomical dead space plus that going to unperfused alveoli and a portion that goes to poorly perfused alveoli (Fig. 4.3). These poorly perfused (or excessively ventilated) areas consist of some perfect alveoli (normal gas exchange) and some unperfused alveoli. Thus the total physiological dead space is not an anatomically identifiable volume, but an effective volume that we obtain by calculation. It reflects the inefficiency of ventilation as it affects CO_2 exchange.

The total expired volume of air per minute comes from two sources: ideal alveoli with $PA_{CO_2} = Pa_{CO_2}$ and unperfused areas (conducting airways or alveolar dead space) with $PI_{CO_2} = 0$, resulting in the physiological dead space relationship (for derivation, see appendix) at the end of this chapter):

$$\frac{V_D}{V_T} = \frac{Pa_{CO_2} - PE_{CO_2}}{Pa_{CO_2}} \tag{4.12}$$

By convention, this is referred to as the V_D/V_T or *wasted fraction* of each tidal breath. Multiplication this fraction by the tidal volume or minute ventilation gives the volume of physiological dead space or wasted ventilation. Dead space thus has the effect of diluting the CO_2 content of expired air below the alveolar level. Because the body needs to expire a certain volume of CO_2 per minute, the effect of a low PE_{CO_2} is to require more total ventilation to maintain homeostasis.

When measuring physiological dead space, one must remember that the volume of air in the mouthpiece, connectors, and valves (mechanical dead space) of the ventilator will also contribute CO_2-free air to the expired air that is collected and measured.

Inspiration of Foreign Substances

Inspired air contains various gases and aerosol particles, many of which are pollutants. The lungs process these inhaled particles and gases in a number of ways, depending on their physical characteristics.

Inhaled Gases

Inhaled gases will be absorbed in either the airways or the alveoli, depending on gas solubility. Gases of very high solubility, such as the alcohols (methyl, ethyl, and butyl), will deposit in the nasopharynx and upper airways. These gases diffuse through the airway tissue and are taken up by the bronchial circulation (see Chapter 5). As gas solubility decreases, the gas penetrates further into the airway tree before being absorbed. The respiratory gases have a relatively low solubility and penetrate the alveoli entirely before being absorbed by the pulmonary circulation blood. The airways are also involved in the uptake of gases that are reactive but not particularly soluble. Pollutant gases, such as ozone (O_3) or sulfur dioxide (SO_2), fall into the latter category.

Inhaled Particles

Inhaled aerosol particles are also taken up at various points within the lungs, depending on their size, but the physical mechanisms of uptake are very different from those of gases. Three major mechanisms have been identified: gravitational settling, inertial impaction, and diffusion. Particle settling due to the pull of gravity occurs with a uniform speed that is proportional to the density of the particle and the square of its diameter. Thus bigger and heavier particles settle more rapidly. When the airstream changes direction, a particle continues in the original direction due to inertia, depending on density and the square of its diameter. If it collides with an airway wall before it can change direction, it is absorbed. Thus larger and heavier particles are more likely to hit the airway walls in the larger airways and nasopharynx. Impaction on the airway wall due to diffusion is caused by normal random motion of the particle.

Figure 4.7 shows the results of experiments that measure the deposition of aerosols of differing size in the nasal cavity, tracheobronchial regions, and the alveoli. Generally speaking, large particles deposit in the nose and upper airways via inertial impaction. Smaller particles pass through the upper airways and deposit

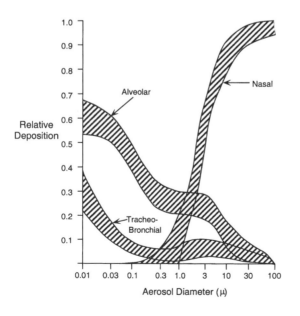

Figure 4.7. Relative deposition of aerosols in three different regions of the respiratory system versus aerosol size. (From Task Group on Lung Dynamics, Committee II. Deposition and retention models for internal dosimetry of the human respiratory tract. *Health Physics* 12:173–208, 1966, with permission.)

in the alveoli via gravitational settling. The very smallest particles diffuse rapidly and are absorbed as soon as they enter in the smaller airways, or the alveoli because of the small diffusion distances. The relative mass of these very small particles is, of course, quite small and not considered important. The very large particles with the greatest mass are deposited in the nose and upper airways, where they are cleared by the mucociliary system. It is the particles between 1 and 5 μm in diameter that are deposited in the alveoli and have sufficient mass to provide a significant dose of pollutant substance.

Appendix

Alveolar Ventilation Equation For Carbon Dioxide

The alveolar ventilation equation for carbon dioxide is

$$\dot{V}_{CO_2} = \dot{V}_A \, FA_{CO_2} = \dot{V}_E \, FE_{CO_2} \tag{4.4}$$

where FA_{CO_2} is the concentration of CO_2 in the alveolar space and FE_{CO_2} is the concentration of CO_2 in mixed expired gas. From this equation, a relationship between PA_{CO_2} and ventilation can be derived.

Rearranging

$$FA_{CO_2} = \frac{\dot{V}_{CO_2}}{\dot{V}_A}$$

and substituting

$$FA_{CO_2} \, (P_B - 47) = PA_{CO_2}$$

we have

$$PA_{CO_2} = \frac{\dot{V}_{CO_2}}{\dot{V}_A} \, (P_B - 47) \tag{4.5}$$

Alveolar Ventilation Equation For Oxygen

The alveolar ventilation equation for O_2 is

$$\dot{V}_{O_2} = \dot{V}_A \, FI_{O_2} - FA_{O_2}$$

or

$$F_{I_{O_2}} - F_{A_{O_2}} = \frac{\dot{V}_{O_2}}{\dot{V}_A}$$

Converting to partial pressure and multiplying both sides by ($P_B - 47$) results in the following:

$$P_{I_{O_2}} - P_{A_{O_2}} = \frac{\dot{V}_{O_2}}{\dot{V}_A} (P_B - 47) \tag{4.8}$$

The alveolar gas exchange equation can be derived as follows by comparing the change in alveolar P_{O_2} and P_{CO_2}:

$$P_{I_{O_2}} - P_{A_{O_2}} = P_{A_{CO_2}}$$

It is clinically useful to us in understanding arterial blood gas values in patients to estimate the $P_{A_{O_2}}$. We see from the discussion above that if $\dot{V}_{CO_2} = \dot{V}_{O_2}$, then (rearranging the previous equation)

$$P_{A_{O_2}} = P_{I_{O_2}} - P_{A_{O_2}}$$

Because the measure of Pa_{CO_2} (arterial P_{CO_2}) is very close to the $P_{A_{CO_2}}$, we can rewrite this equation as follows:

$$P_{A_{O_2}} = P_{I_{O_2}} - Pa_{CO_2}$$

In reality, $\dot{V}_{CO_2}$ and $\dot{V}_{O_2}$ are not necessarily identical but are closely linked with a ratio of $\dot{V}_{CO_2}/\dot{V}_{O_2}$ as the respiratory quotient or respiratory exchange ratio (R).

$$P_{A_{O_2}} = P_{I_{O_2}} - \frac{Pa_{CO_2}}{R}$$

Physiological Dead Space Equation

The total expired volume of air per minute comes from two sources: ideal alveoli with $P_{A_{CO_2}} = Pa_{CO_2}$, and unperfused areas (conducting airways or alveolar dead space) with $P_{I_{CO_2}} = 0$. The total expired volume of CO_2 comes entirely from the effective (non-dead space) alveolar ventilation ($\dot{V}_E - \dot{V}_D$).

$$\dot{V}_{CO_2} = \dot{V}_E \, F_{E_{CO_2}} = (\dot{V}_E - \dot{V}_D) \, F_{A_{CO_2}} + \dot{V}_D \cdot 0$$

Algebraic manipulation yields the following:

$$\dot{V}_D F_{A_{CO_2}} = \dot{V}_E \, F_{A_{CO_2}} - \dot{V}_E F_{E_{CO_2}}$$

$$\frac{V_D}{V_T} = \frac{F_{A_{CO_2}} - F_{E_{CO_2}}}{F_{A_{CO_2}}}$$

Multiplying top and bottom by $(P_B - 47)$ converts the fraction to partial pressure:

$$\frac{V_D}{V_T} = \frac{P_{A_{CO_2}} - P_{E_{CO_2}}}{P_{A_{CO_2}}}$$

Because ideal alveoli with $P_{A_{CO_2}}$ equal to Pa_{CO_2} are assumed, the measured arterial blood gas value can be used, and Pa_{CO_2} is substituted for $P_{A_{CO_2}}$. $P_{E_{CO_2}}$ is obtained from a collection of expired gas:

$$\frac{V_D}{V_T} = \frac{Pa_{CO_2} - P_{E_{CO_2}}}{Pa_{CO_2}} \qquad (4.12)$$

Further Reading

1. Anthonisen NR, Fleetham JA. Ventilation: Total, alveolar, and dead space. In: Farhi LE, Tenney SM, editors. *Handbook of Physiology*, Section 3, *The Respiratory System*, vol IV, *Gas Exchange*. Bethesda, MD: American Physiological Society, 1987, pp 113–130.
2. Kellogg RH. Laws of physics pertaining to gas exchange. In: Farhi LE, Tenney SM, editors. *Handbook of Physiology*, Section 3, *The Respiratory System*, vol IV, *Gas Exchange*. Bethesda, MD: American Physiological Society, 1987, pp 13–32.
3. Scheid P, Piiper J. Diffusion. In: Crystal RG, JB West, ER Weibel, PJ Barns, editors. The Lung: Scientific Foundations, 2nd ed, vol 2. Philadelphia: Lippincott-Raven Publishers,1997, pp 1681–1691.

Study Questions

4.1. Describe how the partial pressures of inspired gases change during the heating and humidification as air passes through the airways.

4.2. Describe both quantitatively and conceptually how alveolar P_{O_2} and P_{CO_2} change with alterations in ventilation. Consider changes in ventilation caused by both exercise and voluntary changes at rest.

4.3. Explain how changes in metabolic respiratory quotient cause changes in $P_{A_{O_2}}$.

4.4. Explain why alveolar P_{N_2} changes during the respiratory cycle.

4.5. What is the physiological dead space ratio in a normal subject with Pa_{CO_2} and PE_{CO_2} values of 40 and 25 mm Hg, respectively? How would you expect the physiological V_D/V_T to change with exercise?

4.6. Where would you expect to find the majority of separate aerosols of 0.03μm, 0.3μm, 3μm, and 30 μm deposited in the respiratory system?

4.7. A patient is being ventilated at a respiratory rate of 10 per minute and a tidal volume of 750 ml. The patient's dead space is 150 ml, and the dead space of the apparatus is also 150 ml.

 A. What is the total ventilation per minute?

   What is the alveolar ventilation?

   What volume change do the alveoli undergo with each breath?

 B. If you collect the expired gas in a bag for 1 minute, what will the P_{CO_2} in the bag be?

4.8. A normal subject is breathing room air and expiring into a large collection bag. When the expired air is analyzed, the mean expired PE_{CO_2} is measured at 30 mm Hg. When the arterial blood is sampled, Pa_{CO_2} is measured at 50 mm Hg. The subject's respiratory frequency is 15 breaths per minute, and the dry gas volume of her average tidal exhalation is 500 ml.

 A. Calculate the physiological dead space fraction.

 B. Calculate the alveolar ventilation.

 C. Calculate the CO_2 production rate.

 Are these values within the normal range?

5

Pulmonary Circulation

The lungs and cardiovascular system work in concert to transport O_2 and CO_2 between the outside environment and the cells of the body. Bringing blood in close proximity to the ventilated air within the lung yields a high degree of gas exchange efficiency. The pulmonary circulation system has special properties that help deliver blood to the alveoli for gas exchange with a very small energy utilization.

In mammals there are two separate circulations in the lung. Pulmonary circulation carries deoxygenated blood to the alveoli for the uptake of O_2 and release of CO_2. This pulmonary circulation carries the entire output of the right heart. In addition, there is a small bronchial circulation (see Chapter 2) that carries systemic arterial blood to the large airways and maintains tissue nutrition if some portion of the pulmonary circulation fails. The bronchial circulation represents only a small fraction (usually about 1% to 2%) of the left ventricular cardiac output. A very important feature of the bronchial circulation is its ability to respond to the need for a long-term increase in regional flow by enlarging vessels or forming new vessels in order to supply areas of the lung that have been damaged by chronic inflammation such as lung abscesses, thrombosis, embolism, stenosis, or arterial ligation.

The Pulmonary Circulation

Blood is driven through the pulmonary vasculature by the pressure difference across any segment. In passing from the right ventricle through the pulmonary blood vessels to the left atrium, blood proceeds along a declining hydrostatic pressure profile. To minimize fluid loss from the pulmonary capillaries to the alveoli or to the extravascular interstitial space, the system maintains a low hydrostatic pressure. The arterioles are relatively narrow and produce most of the resistance (about 80%)

to blood flow in pulmonary circulation. The veins are large and distensible; there is little pressure drop in the veins, even when cardiac output is high. Large veins help capillary hydrostatic pressure remain low due to the low resistance.

The resistance (R) of a blood vessel depends on both the physical dimensions of the vessel and the properties of the blood (see Chapter 1):

$$R = \frac{K \, \ell \eta}{r^4} \qquad (5.1)$$

where K is a constant, ℓ is length, η is viscosity, and r is radius. Resistance depends mainly on vessel radius. Halving of the radius causes a 16-fold increase in resistance. Changes in hematocrit can alter blood viscosity, which in turn can affect vascular resistance, although to a much smaller extent than do changes in vessel radius.

Overall, pulmonary vascular resistance is determined by the resistance of a large number of vessels of various sizes arranged in a complex pattern. Total pulmonary vascular resistance (PVR) is determined by the driving pressure ($\Delta P = P_{pa} - P_{la}$) required to circulate the entire cardiac output ($\dot{Q}$) through the pulmonary system:

$$PVR = \frac{\Delta P}{\dot{Q}} = \frac{P_{pa} - P_{la}}{\dot{Q}} \qquad (5.2)$$

The effective driving pressure for the pulmonary circulation is derived from the difference between pulmonary arterial pressure (P_{pa}) and left atrial pressure (P_{la}). For a given $\dot{Q}$, an increase in ΔP (usually through an increase in P_{pa}) signifies an increase in PVR. Accordingly, a decrease in P_{pa} driving the same cardiac output signifies a decrease in PVR.

A change in ΔP is often misinterpreted as reflective of direct changes in vascular tone. The relationship between ΔP and $\dot{Q}$ is nonlinear (Fig. 5.1) due to changes in the microvasculature that occur with changes in blood flow. The PVR decreases as flow and pressure increase, possibly due to new vessel recruitment. In addition, vascular distention at higher vascular pressures will decrease the resistance of a vessel. As flow decreases, there is a derecruitment of vessels, and this results in an increase in PVR. Changes in PVR with no change in $\dot{Q}$ may reflect vasoconstriction or dilation. Decreases in PVR accompanied by increases in $\dot{Q}$ may, however, simply reflect vascular distension due to increased intravascular pressure.

Blood flows through the pulmonary and systemic circulatory systems in series (see Fig. 1.1). The right heart provides the energy for flow through the pulmonary vasculature, producing a hydrostatic pressure of 25, 6, and 15 mm Hg for systolic,

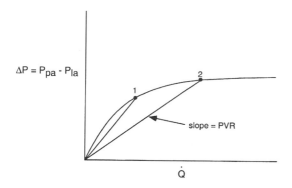

$\Delta P = P_{pa} - P_{la}$

slope = PVR

$\dot{Q}$

Figure 5.1. Driving pressure across the pulmonary circulation ($P_{pa} - P_{la}$) versus cardiac output. Points 1 and 2 represent normal and high cardiac outputs, respectively. The slope of the line connecting each point to the origin refers to pulmonary vascular resistance [($P_{pa} - P_{la})/\dot{Q}$]. The pulmonary vascular resistance (PVR) for point 2 is lower than the PVR for point 1.

diastolic, and mean pressure, respectively. The pressure drops from approximately 13 mm Hg in the arterioles to 9 mm Hg in the pulmonary venules when passing through the pulmonary capillaries. The pressure drop in the pulmonary veins is quite small, reaching a left atrial pressure of 5 mm Hg. The left heart pumps the same amount of blood flow using higher pressures of 120, 80, and 100 mm Hg for systolic, diastolic, and mean pressures, respectively. The pressure decreases through the systemic circulation to a right atrial pressure of about 2 mm Hg. Because the blood flow through both circulations is identical, the relative vascular resistance of the pulmonary and systemic systems can be determined using equation 5.2 (above):

$$\frac{SVR}{PVR} = \frac{\dfrac{(P_{sa} - P_{ra})}{\dot{Q}}}{\dfrac{(P_{pa} - P_{la})}{\dot{Q}}} = \frac{(P_{sa} - P_{ra})}{(P_{pa} - P_{la})} = \frac{(100 - 2)}{(15 - 5)} \approx 10 \qquad (5.3)$$

where P_{sa}, P_{pa}, P_{ra}, and P_{la} are the mean pressures of systemic artery, pulmonary artery, right atrium, and left atrium, respectively. Thus the systemic vascular resistance (SVR) is about 10 times that of the PVR. This is one of the reasons why the right ventricle is less muscular than the left ventricle.

Distribution of Pulmonary Blood Flow

The distribution of blood flow through the lungs plays a critical role in determining the efficiency of pulmonary gas exchange (see Chapter 7). The mechanisms of pulmonary blood flow distribution have been the focus of much research over the past four decades. These mechanisms, however, are not yet fully understood. There are several factors, including vascular structure, gravity, local stresses, and hypoxic pulmonary vasoconstriction, that have an impact on the distribution of blood flow.

Distribution of Pulmonary Blood Flow—Vascular Structure

The major factor influencing pulmonary blood flow distribution is the branching pattern of the blood vessels. At each pulmonary vascular branch point, the flow is directed to each daughter vessel in proportion to the fractional resistance of that vessel. The progressive branching pattern of the blood vessels is similar in geometry at each successive generation, leading to a heterogeneously distributed pulmonary blood flow distribution that depends on the size of the lung pieces used to measure the degree of heterogeneity. This creates a significant heterogeneity within regions that are at the same vertical height in the lung. This regional nonuniformity has been identified with intravascularly injected fluorescent microspheres.

Data from blood flow measurements in small pieces throughout the lungs of a baboon (an animal with lungs that are very similar to those of humans) are shown in Figure 5.2 plotted against the vertical height of the lung in the erect (head-up) position. In the erect position, blood flow is greatest in the bottom (caudal) regions of the lungs and lowest in the top (cranial) regions. At any given height up the lung (except at the very top), there is considerable variation of blood flow within any isogravitational plane (regions at a given height from the bottom of the lung). The regression line in Figure 5.2 indicates a vertical gradient in average blood flow. The blood flow within individual small regions remains relatively constant from time to time and with exercise or changes in posture. In the prone posture, there is only a negligible vertical gradient in average blood flow while the variability in the horizontal plane remains. The blood flow in adjacent regions is highly correlated (high flow pieces are near high flow pieces and low flow pieces are near low flow pieces), indicating that local flow may be determined by the resistance of arteriolar vessels feeding the region. Thus, the orientation of the gravity vector relative to the rib cage, diaphragm, and abdominal contents influences the relative importance of vascular structure relative to that of gravity.

Distribution of Pulmonary Blood Flow—Gravity

In the 1960s, physiologists developed a model focusing on gravitational force of the earth as a dominant factor in determining the distribution of pulmonary blood flow. This idea considers the hydrostatic pressure in blood vessels to be governed by the vertical height of the blood vessel. The implicit assumption is that there is no viscous energy loss within the pulmonary arteries and arterioles. Local pulmonary vascular resistance and local pulmonary flow were thought to be influenced by the difference between intravascular and extravascular pressures. Extravascular

Erect (Upright) Position

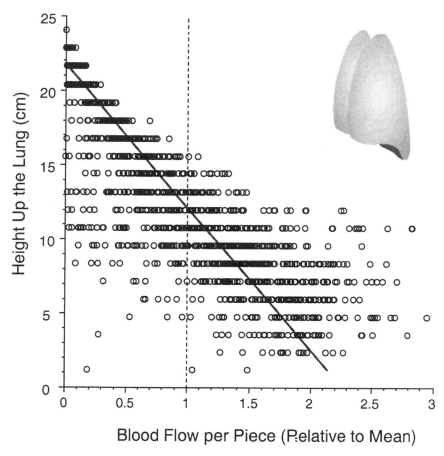

Figure 5.2. Vertical distribution of blood flow in the baboon lung in the erect posture. Considerable heterogeneity of blood flow is seen within each isogravitational plane. (From Glenny RW et al. Gravity is an important but secondary determinant of regional pulmonary blood flow in upright primates. *J Appl Physiol* 86:623–632, 1999.)

pressure is closely related to alveolar pressure, which is near zero (relative to atmospheric pressure)—with the exception of small variations during inspiration and expiration—and is similar throughout the lung. Intravascular pressure, on the other hand, varies significantly at different points of lung height due to the influence of gravity.

Local pulmonary arterial pressure depends on the pulmonary artery pressure (measured at the height of the right atrium, the zero reference point for the pulmonary circulation) minus the pressure difference of the hydrostatic column of blood between the point of interest and the height of the left atrium. Normal values for systolic and diastolic pulmonary pressures are

$$\frac{25 \text{ mm Hg}}{6 \text{ mm Hg}} \times \frac{1.36 \dfrac{\text{cm H}_2\text{O}}{\text{mm Hg}}}{1.36 \dfrac{\text{cm H}_2\text{O}}{\text{mm Hg}}} = \frac{34 \text{ cm H}_2\text{O} \text{ (systolic)}}{8 \text{ cm H}_2\text{O} \text{ (diastolic)}} \qquad (5.4)$$

In arteries below the left atrium, the pressure is greater. In an artery that is about 5 cm lower than the left atrium, the arterial pressure will be approximately 5cm H_2O higher (or systolic and diastolic pressures of 39 and 13cm H_2O, respectively). Progressing upward in the lungs, the pulmonary arterial pressure decreases. P_{pa} would eventually reach zero at a point 34 cm above the left atrium, which would be above the top of the lungs. Zero flow regions due to zero arterial pressure do not exist in the normal human lung. These relationships have led to the zone model (Fig. 5.3) of the pulmonary vascular system.

The zone model predicts that zone 1, which might occur at the top of the lung, is characterized by an arterial pressure that falls to zero. Above this point, the vascular pressure is not sufficient to perfuse the alveolar vessels, and they remain collapsed. Alveolar pressure exceeds both pulmonary arterial pressure and pulmonary venous pressure ($P_A > P_a > P_v$) in this region. Zone 1 does not exist

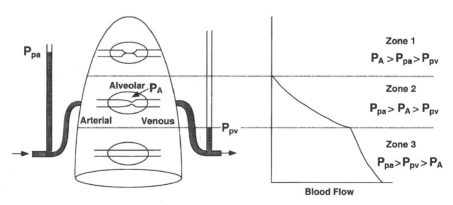

Figure 5.3. The zone model. Flow is a function of vertical height and is dependent on the relationship between alveolar and vascular pressures. (From Hlastala MP, Glenny RW. Vascular structure determines pulmonary blood flow distribution. *News Physiol Sci* 14:182–186, 1999.)

in normal human lungs because the left atrium is close enough to the top of the lung to maintain a positive intravascular pressure. If pulmonary arterial pressure decreases for some reason, such as a reduced cardiac output, conditions for a zone 1 region may develop.

In zone 2, pulmonary arterial pressure exceeds alveolar pressure, allowing capillary perfusion. As blood flow proceeds through the capillaries, intravascular pressure decreases, eventually reaching the point where it is lower than alveolar pressure. This results in a compressive force on the pulmonary capillaries, decreasing the intravascular cross-sectional area and increasing resistance. Intravascular pressure then declines rapidly to equal venous pressure, which is lower than alveolar pressure in zone 2 ($P_a > P_A > P_v$). In zone 2, flow depends on the difference in driving pressure between P_a and P_A and is unaffected by venous pressure. This is analogous to a waterfall where the flow depends on the gradient above the fall and is not affected by the height of the fall. With progression from zone 1 down into zone 2, both P_a and ($P_a - P_A$) increase, resulting in an increase in flow.

In zone 3, vascular pressure always exceeds alveolar pressure ($P_a > P_v > P_A$). Here, the capillaries remain open, and flow depends on the difference between P_a and P_v. With changes in height within zone 3, P_a and P_v change together. Thus ($P_a - P_v$) is constant within zone 3. With progression from zone 2 down into zone 3, overall vascular pressures rise, causing increased transcapillary pressure, increased capillary size, and therefore lower resistance. Thus, flow continues to increase with descent into zone 3.

The observation of a region of reduced blood flow near the bottom of the lungs led some investigators to hypothesize the presence of a zone 4 (not shown in Fig. 5.3). This region of reduced flow has been thought to be due to either a compression of the lung parenchyma and increased vascular resistance or development of interstitial edema due to increased hydrostatic pressure in the vasculature in the bottom of the lung leading to increased vascular resistance and decreased flow. The finding that blood flow in the caudal regions (near the diaphragm) of the lung remains low even when the vertical orientation of the lungs is reversed, however, argues against this gravity-dependent explanation of zone 4.

Recent studies based on high spatial resolution methods have demonstrated that gravity is only a minor influence on the regional distribution of pulmonary blood flow in the mammal.

Fractal Analysis

The observed blood flow distribution in mammalian lungs can be analyzed by using fractal analysis. Fractal structures are composed of successively smaller parts, each of which is similar to the whole. There is a constant pattern (such as a bifurcating one) that repeats itself at each branch generation. If the resulting blood flow to each vascular generation is uneven, the degree of overall variation will increase as the size of the individual units measured decreases. If the flow to each piece is assessed by the coefficient of variation (CV, which is the standard deviation/mean), then the CV increases as resolution increases (piece size decreases). Figure 5.4 shows the relationship between coefficient of variation of pulmonary blood flow heterogeneity versus the size of the pieces of lung. Six different lungs are shown. Each has a different CV at the minimum piece size (V_0). The slopes of the lines of regression (indicating the change in CV with change in piece size) are similar for each lung.

The fractal dimension (D_s) can be determined from the slope (s): (D_s = 1 − s) of the regression line of ln (CV) versus ln (piece size) (Fig. 5.4). When D_s = 1, the system is scale independent. D_s = 1.5 represents random heterogeneity. For the lungs shown in Figure 5.4, D_s ranged between 1.07 and 1.12, with an average of 1.09. This indicates that the flow heterogeneity is not random, but is largely dependent on the fractal branching pattern of the pulmonary vasculature.

Contrary to predictions of the zone model, there is a high degree of similarity in flow to adjacent pieces. When the relative similarity of flow to any given piece is compared with the variation in flow among different positions, variance analysis shows that gravity (the zone model) accounts for less than 25% of the variation shown in Figure 5.2. Most of the variation in blood flow distribution is related to local pulmonary vascular branching and other anatomical factors.

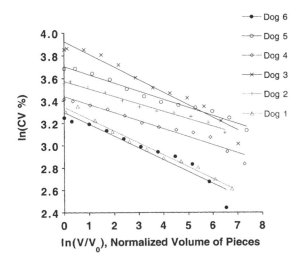

Figure 5.4. Coefficient of variation (CV) of normalized regional pulmonary blood flows plotted as a function of volume of aggregated lung pieces. For each animal, the individual data points are shown for the CV for each piece size. Regression lines for each animal are shown. (From Glenny RW et al. Applications of fractal analysis to physiology. *J Appl Physiol* 70:2351–2367, 1970.)

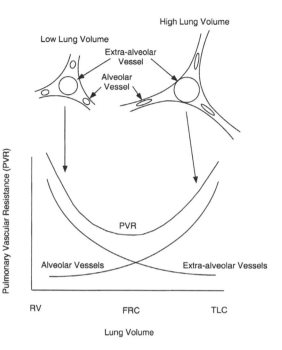

Figure 5.5. Pulmonary vascular resistance versus lung volume. Overall vascular resistance is made up of resistances of both alveolar vessels (capillaries) and extraalveolar vessels (arterioles and venules). Increasing lung volume causes an enlargement of extraalveolar vessels and a compression of alveolar vessels. Overall vascular resistance increases at low lung volume due to a decrease in the size of the extraalveolar vessels and increases at high lung volume due to a decrease in the size of the alveolar vessels.

Local Stresses

Superimposed on the gravity-dependent perfusion distribution are local stresses that alter vascular resistance. Increasing lung volume stretches and distends extraalveolar arterial and venous vessels. However, lung inflation also causes elongation and compression of capillaries within alveolar walls, so-called alveolar vessels. The resistances of both alveolar and extraalveolar vessels are in series and therefore additive. This result is an increased pulmonary vascular resistance (decreased flow) with either lung inflation or deflation from FRC (Fig. 5.5).

The relative amount of change in vascular resistance with lung volume is influenced by the differences of expansion of the relatively rigid airways and relatively compliant parenchyma. During lung expansion, blood vessels within parenchyma near the airways are distorted, resulting in local changes in local vascular resistance.

Hypoxic Vasoconstriction

The pulmonary vasculature is regulated by alveolar gases in a manner that helps to normalize the matching of $\dot{V}_A/\dot{Q}$ and makes gas exchange more efficient. The smaller arterioles constrict when local alveolar P_{O_2} falls (Fig. 5.6). This constriction is augmented if alveolar P_{CO_2} rises. Hypoxic vasoconstriction is a response to a decrease of the P_{O_2} in the alveolar gas, not in the blood, causing hypoxic vasoconstriction only in those regions that are hypoxic. When ventilation is decreased by an obstructed airway or other injury, local hypoxic vasoconstriction reduces local blood flow. Thus the ventilation/perfusion ratio ($\dot{V}_A/\dot{Q}$) of these regions stays close to normal, despite decreased local ventilation, and gas exchange remains near normal (see Chapter 7). In patients with generalized alveolar hypoxia due to lung disease or low $P_{I_{O_2}}$ (altitude), elevated pulmonary vascular resistance and eventual right heart failure may result. At high altitude, some normal individuals develop high altitude pulmonary edema (HAPE), possibly because of a greater hypoxic vasoconstriction response that causes elevated vascular pressure (see Fig. 11.4).

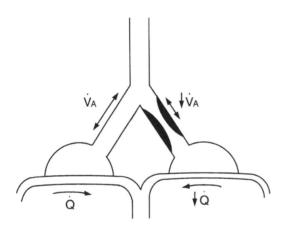

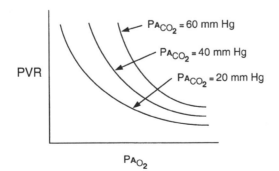

Figure 5.6. Pulmonary vascular resistance is plotted against $P_{A_{O_2}}$. Curves for three different $P_{A_{CO_2}}$ values are shown. The upper schematic shows an alveolus with reduced ventilation due to bronchial constriction. Hypoxic vasoconstriction reduces the blood flow to that alveolus, returning its $\dot{V}_A/\dot{Q}$ to normal.

Fluid Exchange by the Pulmonary Circulation

Fluid is exchanged continually between the pulmonary vessels and the interstitium and between the interstitium and the pleural space. This fluid exchange is well regulated to prevent accumulation of excessive fluid in either the interstitium or the pleural space. This normal exchange is governed by a balance between hydrostatic and oncotic pressure differences. There is a small net fluid loss to the interstitium that is taken up in the lymphatic system, which prevents the accumulation of excess fluid. The precise location of fluid filtration from the intravascular space to the interstitial space is not known, but about 60% of this filtration occurs in alveolar capillaries, about 15% occurs in the extraalveolar arterial vessels, and about 25% occurs in the extraalveolar venous vessels.

Fluid movement across the pulmonary capillaries has been described by the *Starling relationship*:

$$J_W = K_f \left[\left(P_{mv} - P_{isf} \right) - \sigma \left(\pi_p - \pi_{isf} \right) \right] \tag{5.5}$$

where J_w is net fluid flux across the vessel wall, K_f is capillary filtration coefficient, σ is osmotic reflection coefficient, P_{mv} is pressure in microvessels, P_{isf} is perimicrovascular tissue pressure, π_p is plasma osmotic pressure, and π_{isf} is interstitial fluid osmotic pressure. The net filtration pressure refers to the difference in hydrostatic pressure between the microvessel and the surrounding tissue, which results in a net outward filtration. The net absorption pressure, the difference between the osmotic pressure of the plasma and the surrounding interstitial space, results in a net inward absorption. The difference between filtration and absorption pressures determines the direction of fluid movement, and K_f refers to the ease of fluid movement.

Intravascular hydrostatic pressure is determined by the balance of precapillary and postcapillary resistances. Normally, the arterial segment has the greatest resistance; thus capillary pressure is much closer to left atrial than to pulmonary arterial pressure. If the venous resistance rises for some reason (venous constriction or perivenous cuffing), however, or if left atrial pressure rises (as in congestive heart failure), the capillary pressure will rise, increasing the driving force for filtering fluid.

A positive interstitial hydrostatic fluid pressure opposes filtration. The pulmonary interstitial fluid pressure is normally subatmospheric (negative relative to left atrial pressure) because of lymphatic drainage and the recoil pressure of the lung, thus enhancing filtration. Some fluid always moves from the alveolar capillaries into the perivascular spaces to be removed by the lymphatic vessels. The fluid exiting the alveolar capillaries is filtered through a dense basement membrane and the interstitium, which contains extracellular fluid, mucopolysaccharides, and collagen. The normal pressure surrounding the alveolar vessels is believed to be about 1 to 2 mm Hg higher than that in the perivascular space. The alveolo-capillary membrane has little compliance and swells only slightly when interstitial fluid begins to accumulate. Large amounts of fluid move rapidly into the more compliant perivascular spaces, which can accommodate large volumes of fluid with only small changes in pressure. After large amounts of fluid exceed the capacity of the lymphatics, fluid moves from the interstitium to the alveolar space, and alveolar edema develops.

Proteins in liquid exert a colloid osmotic (or oncotic) pressure. In the plasma, protein moves fluid from the tissues into the capillaries. In the interstitial space, protein tends to pull fluid from the plasma into the interstitial space. The protein concentration in plasma is greater than that in the interstitial space, causing a net absorptive force that counteracts the net filtration force of the hydrostatic pressure difference. Albumin is the major protein in plasma (4 to 5 gm $\cdot$ dl^{-1}), whereas α_2-, β-, and γ-globulins together comprise about 3 gm $\cdot$ dl^{-1} of the total 7.5 gm $\cdot$ dl^{-1} plasma protein concentration, exerting an osmotic pressure of 28 mm Hg. The plasma protein concentration in the interstitium is about 4 to 5 gm $\cdot$ dl^{-1} and exerts an osmotic pressure of 15 to 20 mm Hg.

The permeability of the capillary wall, as indicated by the value of K_f, has several determining factors, including the total exchange surface area, the number of pores through which fluid can move contained within this area, and the radius of these pores to the fourth power. Thus K_f defines the amount of fluid that crosses the capillary wall for a given difference between the filtration and absorptive forces.

The relative balance of the filtration and absorption forces changes dynamically. Because fluid leaking from blood is largely protein free, it dilutes the interstitial protein concentration. This reduces perivascular π_{isf}, increasing the inward osmotic pressure difference (particularly because the filtration of water causes blood π_{mv} to rise) and reduces the local fluid leak. If excess leakage occurs, fluid shifts from the interstitium to the space surrounding the bronchioles and arterioles, where it forms relatively innocuous venous, arterial, and peribronchial cuffs (fluid constricting vessel size and increasing resistance). This fluid is absorbed by a rich bronchial vascular network and by the many lymphatics in the adventitia of the airways and vessels. Edema fluid is also shifted into the pleural space to be absorbed by the lymphatic and systemic pleural blood vessels.

When fluid filtering exceeds the capacity of lymphatics to return the fluid to the circulation and the peribronchial and perivascular cuffs reach maximum volume, the alveolar epithelial cells tear and alveolar edema ensues. Figure 5.7 shows the pulmonary capillary structure with interstitial edema. Note the marked

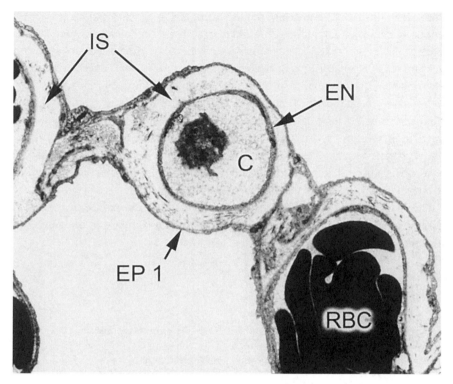

Figure 5.7. Transmission electron micrograph of the alveolar capillary region after development of interstitial edema. C, Capillary; EN, capillary endothelial cell; EP 1, alveolar type I epithelial cell; IS, interstitial space; RBC, erythrocyte. (Adapted from Velazquez M et al. PET evaluation of pulmonary vascular permeability: A structure–function correlation. *J Appl Physiol* 70:2206–2216, 1991.)

widening of the interstitial space (IS) compared with the thin IS in the normal lungs (see Fig. 2.8).

Pulmonary edema is a potentially serious problem in diseases that increase pulmonary vascular hydrostatic pressure, such as pulmonary hypertension, or increase vascular permeability, such as in adult respiratory distress syndrome (ARDS).

Pulmonary Blood Flow During Breathing

Because the pulmonary circulation is located within the thorax with its changing pressure, fluctuations in blood flow during the respiratory cycle ensue. With inspiration, the fall in pleural pressure reduces right atrial pressure and hence increases venous return. Capillary blood flow increases at the onset of inhalation but then tends to fall as vascular resistance increases with lung volume. Pulmonary arterial pressure remains relatively constant while left atrial pressure falls. Due to the surrounding negative intrapleural pressure, the emptying of intrapulmonary veins may be limited by a pulmonary venous waterfall (similar to that in zone 2) where the veins exit from the lung parenchyma.

During expiration, an increase in pleural pressure decreases systemic venous return and hence right heart output. As lung volume decreases, events opposing those during inspiration occur. In addition, the rise in pericardial pressure (relative to atmospheric) increases the pressure surrounding the left ventricle and, thus, systemic arterial pressure. These events contribute to the paradoxical pulse, an increase in systemic pressure during exhalation and a decrease in pressure during inhalation.

Further Reading

1. Culver BH, Butler J. Mechanical influences on the pulmonary microcirculation. *Annu Rev Physiol* 42:187–198, 1980.
2. Dawson CA. Role of pulmonary vasomotion in physiology of the lung. *Physiol Rev* 64: 544–616, 1984.
3. Deffebach ME, Charan NB, Lakshminarayan S, Butler J. The bronchial circulation: Small, but a vital attribute of the lung. *Am Rev Respir Dis* 135:463–481, 1987.
4. Fishman AP. Hypoxia on the pulmonary circulation: How and where it acts. *Circ Res* 38:221–231, 1976.
5. Hughes, JMB. Distribution of pulmonary blood flow. In: Crystal RG, JB West, ER Weibel, PJ Barns, editors, *The Lung: Scientific Foundations*, 2nd ed, vol 2. Philadelphia: Lippincot-Raven Publishers, 1997, pp 1523–1536.
6. Swenson ER, Domino KD, Hlastala MP. Physiological effects of oxygen and carbon dioxide on $\dot{V}_A/\dot{Q}$ Heterogeneity. In: Hlastala MP, Robertson HT, editors. *Lung Biology in Health and Disease,* vol. 121, *Complexity in Structure and Function of the Lung.* MP New York: Marcel Dekker, Inc. 1998, pp 511–547.

Study Questions

5.1. Assume that a normal aortic blood pressure is 120 mm Hg/80 mm Hg (systolic over diastolic). Compute the relative resistance of the pulmonary circulation compared with the systemic circulation.

5.2. Describe the influence of gravity on the distribution of pulmonary blood flow. Include an explanation of the four-zone model and a discussion of experimental observations.

5.3. How does hypoxic pulmonary vasoconstriction help to maintain a normal regional $\dot{V}_A/\dot{Q}$ ratio in response to changes in airway resistance?

5.4. Describe the factors affecting the formation of pulmonary edema.

5.5. Describe how ventilation with positive end-expired pressure (which increases lung volume throughout the ventilatory cycle) would influence pulmonary vascular resistance and pulmonary arterial pressure.

6

Blood Gas Transport and
Tissue Gas Exchange

Storage and transport of O_2 and CO_2 in blood are accomplished by special mechanisms. Hemoglobin is instrumental to the storage of both O_2 and CO_2 in a way that is interactive, a feature that enhances the exchange of each gas and provides a reserve when O_2 demand increases.

Oxygen Transport

Like inert gases, O_2 dissolves in blood in direct proportion to its partial pressure. This relationship is described by *Henry's law*:

$$C_{O_2} = \beta b_{O_2} \, P_{O_2} \qquad (6.1)$$

The proportionality constant relating O_2 content (C_{O_2}) to O_2 partial pressure (P_{O_2}) is βb_{O_2}, the blood solubility coefficient, commonly expressed as ml gas (STPD) dissolved in 100 ml (1 dl) blood for every mm Hg of partial pressure. The value of βb_b differs for each gas (O_2 and CO_2) and varies with temperature. More gas dissolves in liquid as temperature decreases. For blood at 37°C, βb_{O_2} is approximately equal to 0.003 ml $\cdot$ dl^{-1} $\cdot$ mm Hg^{-1}. This low solubility allows only a small portion of O_2 to be dissolved in blood at physiological partial pressures (80 to 100 mm Hg). At a normal arterial P_{O_2} of 100 mm Hg, only 0.3 ml O_2 can be stored as dissolved gas in each dl of blood. This does not, however, meet normal metabolic demands. This requirement is met by hemoglobin with its high O_2 storage capability.

Hemoglobin

Hemoglobin (Hb) is a complex molecule (molecular weight of approximately 64,500) composed primarily of four polypeptide chains. In normal adult humans, Hb has two α-chains (141 amino acids) and two β-chains (146 amino acids). Each polypeptide chain has a heme group that contains an iron atom capable of binding O_2. Each Hb molecule can carry four O_2 molecules. For each gram of Hb, 1.39 ml of O_2 can be stored:

$$4 \, \frac{\text{moles } O_2}{\text{mole Hb}} \times 22{,}400 \, \frac{\text{ml } O_2}{\text{mole } O_2} \times 1 \, \frac{\text{mole Hb}}{64{,}500 \text{ gm Hb}} = 1.39 \, \frac{\text{ml } O_2}{\text{gm Hb}} \quad (6.2)$$

In actuality, fully saturated Hb carries up to 1.34 to 1.36 ml of O_2 per gram because a small fraction of the heme sites cannot bind O_2, largely because a small fraction of the iron on the heme sites that bind O_2 is converted from the ferrous

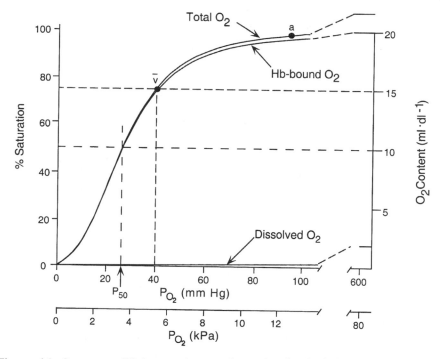

Figure 6.1. Oxygen equilibrium curves are shown for dissolved O_2, hemoglobin-bound O_2, and total O_2 content versus P_{O_2}. The saturation ordinate refers only to hemoglobin-bound O_2. The content ordinate applies to all three curves. a, arterial point; $\bar{v}$, mixed venous points.

form ($^{+++}$) to the ferric form ($^{+++}$) (also called methemoglobin), which cannot bind O_2.

As each O_2 molecule binds to Hb, it increases the affinity of the remaining heme sites for additional O_2 molecules. This is known as *heme–heme interaction* and results in a nonlinear, S shape for the O_2 binding curve, which is called the *oxygen equilibrium* or *dissociation curve* (Fig. 6.1). Because the amount of Hb-bound oxygen is much greater than the amount of dissolved O_2, the total blood O_2 content curve is close to the Hb-bound O_2 content curve.

The shape of the O_2 equilibrium curve has much physiological significance. For high P_{O_2} (in the arterial range), the curve is nearly flat as the Hb approaches saturation and most heme sites bind an O_2 molecule. In the face of mild arterial hypoxemia (decreased P_{O_2}), the O_2 content of blood will remain near maximum. This means that arterial blood can deliver a normal amount of O_2 even with mild respiratory disease or ascent to high altitude, both of which can result in a decreased Pa_{O_2}. As O_2 is delivered to the tissues, the C_{O_2} and P_{O_2} both decrease along the O_2 equilibrium curve. Because this curve is steep and S shaped, a large variation in venous O_2 content can occur while a relatively high P_{O_2} is maintained. It is important that venous (end-capillary) P_{O_2} remain as high as possible to provide sufficient driving force for O_2 diffusion from the capillary to the cell most distant from the capillary, ensuring enough O_2 diffusion to provide the cell's metabolic needs. These needs may vary considerably from moment to moment.

Factors Affecting Hemoglobin–Oxygen Affinity

The relative Hb–O_2 affinity can be characterized by the P_{50} (Fig. 6.1), or the O_2 partial pressure at which Hb is 50% saturated. When O_2 affinity changes, the position of the equilibrium curve and hence the P_{50} change (Fig. 6.2). Increased O_2 affinity corresponds to a leftward shift of the curve and decreased P_{50}; that is, 50% Hb saturation can be achieved at a lower P_{O_2}. Another way to view the leftward shift is that a greater amount of O_2 is bound to Hb at any P_{O_2}. A decreased O_2 affinity corresponds to a rightward shift and increased $P_{50;}$ 50% Hb saturation is now achieved at a higher P_{O_2}.

Hydrogen Ion

Hydrogen ion (H^+) also binds to Hb. This binding occurs at many sites and predominantly with the imidazole group of the amino acid histidine. Increased H^+ (decreased pH) increases H^+ binding to Hb, decreases O_2 affinity (Fig. 6.2), and causes a rightward shift of the O_2 equilibrium curve.

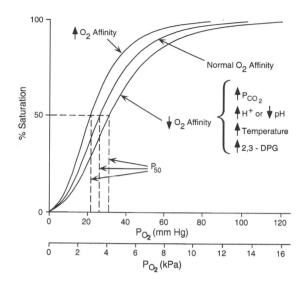

Figure 6.2. Changes in O_2 affinity of the O_2 saturation curve. Three curves are shown with progressively decreasing O_2 affinity indicated by increasing P_{50}.

Carbon Dioxide

Increased P_{CO_2} reduces O_2 affinity. This was first described by Christian Bohr in 1904 and is now known as the *Bohr effect*. This effect is due in part to direct CO_2 binding at the N-terminal valines of both the α- and β-chains. The other cause of the decreased O_2 affinity is the CO_2 hydration reaction:

$$CO_2 + H_2O \xleftrightarrow{\ CA\ } H_2CO_3 \leftrightarrow H^+ + HCO_3^- \qquad (6.3)$$

The H^+ produced binds to Hb, reducing O_2 affinity. These two components of the CO_2 Bohr effect are now differentiated into the CO_2 effect and the fixed-acid Bohr effect. Under normal conditions in adult human blood, these two components have an equal share in the total Bohr effect, although their relative magnitudes can change with various blood acid–base conditions.

Temperature

Temperature also has an important affect on O_2 affinity. Increased temperature reduces O_2 affinity. Although temperature also affects the magnitude of both the CO_2 Bohr effect and the fixed-acid Bohr effect, it is thought that the direct temperature effect on O_2 affinity plays the most important role in matching O_2 delivery with O_2 demand. Increasing temperature increases the metabolic rate, which increases

O_2 demand. The increased O_2 delivery provided by a rightward shift in the O_2 equilibrium curve with increased temperature helps to meet the increased O_2 demand.

2,3-Diphosphoglycerate

2,3-Diphosphoglycerate (DPG) is an intermediate metabolite in the red cell gly-colytic pathway that affects Hb–O_2 affinity. DPG binds to the β-chains within the central cavity of the Hb molecule, decreasing O_2 affinity. Intraerythrocytic acidosis, which may be caused by blood storage in acid-citrate-dextrose solution, will reduce the activity of phosphofructokinase, decreasing DPG concentration and increasing O_2 affinity. Reduced DPG increases Hb–O_2 affinity, but also increases the impor-tance of the CO_2 Bohr effect due to the competitive interaction of DPG and CO_2 at the N-terminal value of the β-chains. Changes in DPG may play a role in ad-aptation to high altitude (see Chapter 11).

Carbon Monoxide

Carbon monoxide (CO) and O_2 bind reversibly to the same site on the Hb molecule. Binding of CO prevents O_2 binding. Because Hb has an affinity for CO that is about 250 times greater than that for O_2, it takes a small amount of CO to displace O_2 from the heme-binding site. CO binding not only decreases the O_2 content but also increases the Hb–O_2 affinity of the remaining heme sites. The resulting O_2 equilibrium curve is reduced in magnitude as well as shifted left (Fig. 6.3). The venous P_{O_2} is reduced due to both a lower O_2 content and a higher Hb–O_2 affinity.

Carbon monoxide is present in the blood at low levels (COHb = 1% to 2%), owing to the normal breakdown of Hb. It is also present at high levels in cigarette smoke and automobile exhaust. The uptake of CO by humans is slow (see Chapter 7), taking between 4 and 8 hours to reach equilibrium. Inspired CO of 100 parts per million (comparable with air near a busy freeway) raises carboxyhemoglobin (COHb) levels to about 14% (also common in heavy smokers). Chronic exposure at this level has long-term effects on the health of smokers and can have direct effects on the babies of smoking mothers. The affinity of fetal Hb for CO is about 50% greater than that of maternal Hb. Higher level exposure (as with smoke in-halation in fires or propane burner accidents) is often treated with 100% O_2 breathing, which reduces the CO washout half-time to 1 hour from 4 hours with air breathing. In a hyperbaric chamber, a patient breathing 100% O_2 will reduce the washout half-time even further while increasing P_{O_2} enough to add a significant amount of dissolved O_2 (about 2.3 ml · dl^{-1} · atmosphere^{-1}) to arterial blood.

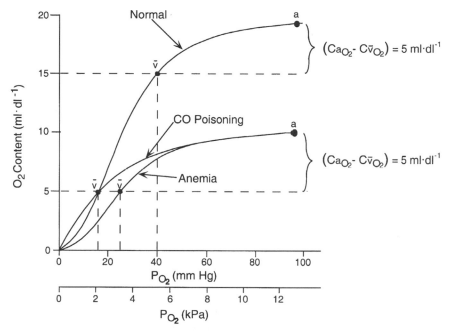

Figure 6.3. Effect of CO and anemia on the O_2 equilibrium curve. Curves are shown for normal blood with Hb = 15 gm · dl^{-1}; anemia with Hb = 7.5 gm · dl^{-1}; and normal blood with 50% COHb. With a normal arterial point (a) and a normal $Ca_{O_2} - C\bar{v}_{O_2}$ difference of 5 ml · dl^{-1}, the mixed venous point ($\bar{v}$) decreased from 40 to 25 to 17 mm Hg for normal, anemia, and COHb curves, respectively.

Anemia

Anemia is a reduction of Hb concentration. The O_2 equilibrium is reduced in O_2 content of Hb at any partial pressure in proportion to the reduction in Hb concentration (see Eq. 6.4). With anemia, a normal cardiac output and arterial–venous oxygen extraction leads to a reduced tissue venous P_{O_2} (see Fig. 6.3).

Arterial and Venous O_2 Content

Within the alveolus, O_2 reaches equilibrium between alveolar gas and pulmonary capillary blood under normal conditions irrespective of Hb concentration. Arterial P_{O_2} is closely tied to alveolar P_{O_2}. Arterial O_2 content is directly related to Hb concentration (Hb) and Hb saturation (Sa_{O_2}) by the following expression:

$$Ca_{O_2} = \text{Portion bound to Hb} + \text{Portion in physical solution}$$

$$Ca_{O_2} = [Hb] \times 1.36 \frac{ml\ O_2}{gm\ Hb} \times Sa_{O_2} + \beta b_{O_2} \times Pa_{O_2} \qquad (6.4)$$

Under normal conditions of arterial blood, $Pa_{O_2} = 100$ mm Hg, $\beta b_{O_2} = 0.003$ ml $\cdot$ dl^{-1} $\cdot$ mm Hg^{-1}, Sa_{O_2} (O_2 saturation) $= 0.97$, and $[Hb] = 15$ gm $\cdot$ dl^{-1}; normal $Ca_{O_2} = 20$ ml $\cdot$ dl^{-1}. Blood with reduced Hb concentration (anemia) retains less O_2, whereas blood with increased Hb concentration (polycythemia) retains more.

Mixed venous O_2 content is determined by the balance between O_2 consumption and cardiac output, as described by the Fick principle:

$$\dot{V}_{O_2} = \dot{Q}\left(Ca_{O_2} - Cv_{O_2}\right) \qquad (6.5)$$

which is derived from the principle of conservation of mass. Uptake of O_2 by blood in the lungs ($\dot{V}_{O_2}$) is equal to the rate of O_2 carried away in arterial blood ($\dot{Q}$ Ca_{O_2}) minus the rate of O_2 returned to the lungs by venous blood ($\dot{Q}$ Cv_{O_2}). Once the venous O_2 content is known, the Pv_{O_2} is determined by using the O_2 equilibrium curve (Fig. 6.1). Typical values for the variables in equation 6.5 are $\dot{V}_{O_2} = 250$ ml $\cdot$ min^{-1}, $\dot{Q} = 5$ l $\cdot$ min^{-1} or 5000 ml $\cdot$ min^{-1}, and $Ca_{O_2} = 20$ ml $\cdot$ dl^{-1} or 0.20 ml $\cdot$ ml^{-1}, which yields a typical venous O_2 content of 0.15 ml $\cdot$ ml^{-1} or 15 ml $\cdot$ dl^{-1}. A content of 15 ml $\cdot$ dl^{-1} in Figure 6.1 indicates Pv_{O_2} of 40 mm Hg. The arterio-venous O_2 content difference is determined by the ratio of $\dot{V}_{O_2}$ to $\dot{Q}$ (Eq 6.5). If $\dot{V}_{O_2}$ decreases or increases, the anteriovenous O_2 difference will decrease and both Cv_{O_2} and Pv_{O_2} will increase. The reverse occurs with an increase in $\dot{V}_{O_2}$ or a decrease in $\dot{Q}$. The $\dot{V}_{O_2}/\dot{Q}$ ratio varies among different organs, that is, venous P_{O_2} of the kidney is normally much higher than venous P_{O_2} of the heart.

Carbon Dioxide Transport

Carbon dioxide is stored in blood in three forms and in a more complex manner than O_2. These forms are physical solution, carbamino (protein bound), and bicarbonate.

The solubility of CO_2 in blood is about 24 times greater than the solubility of O_2, and this enhances storage in the dissolved form. The amount of CO_2 dissolved in arterial blood is

$$C_{CO_2} = \beta_{CO_2}\ P_{CO_2} \qquad (6.6)$$

$$= 0.072\ \frac{ml}{dl \cdot mm\ Hg} \times 40\ mm\ Hg$$

$$= 2.9\ \frac{ml}{dl}$$

This amount represents only 6% of the total arterial CO_2 content under normal conditions.

The second form of storage combines CO_2 with blood proteins. Hemoglobin (carbamino) is by far the greatest quantity of protein participating. Carbon dioxide binds reversibly at the N terminus of both the α-and β-chains of Hb. The carbamino compound reaction releases a proton:

$$R - NH_2 + CO_2 \leftrightarrow R - NH - COO^- + H^+ \qquad (6.7)$$

At normal arterial P_{O_2}, CO_2 stored as carbamino compounds amounts to 2.1 ml · dl^{-1}, or about 4% of the total CO_2 content. Formation of carbamino compounds weakens the O_2 binding affinity of Hb. Conversely, carbamino formation falls when P_{O_2} rises. Even though carbamino makes up only a small fraction of total blood CO_2 storage, it contributes markedly to the change in CO_2 content between venous and arterial blood, accounting for approximately 40% of the CO_2 exchange in the lung or other tissues under normal conditions.

The vast majority of CO_2 storage is in the form of bicarbonate (HCO_3^-). CO_2 rapidly combines with water to form carbonic acid and then rapidly dissociates into hydrogen ion and bicarbonate ion. The first hydration reaction (Eq. 6.3) is catalyzed by carbonic anhydrase within the red cell. The amount of CO_2 stored as bicarbonate in normal arterial blood is about 42 ml · dl^{-1} at a P_{CO_2} of 40 mm Hg. This accounts for the remaining 90% of the total CO_2 storage in the blood.

The impact of O_2 on CO_2 content is termed the *Haldane effect;* increasing O_2 saturation reduces CO_2 content, shifting the CO_2 equilibrium curve to the right (Fig. 6.4). This effect is due in part to the decrease in carbamino and in part to the release of H^+ from hemoglobin and the resulting dehydration of HCO_3^- (Eq. 6.3).

The relative proportion of each storage mechanism changes during capillary transit (Fig. 6.5). In the systemic capillary, CO_2 diffuses from tissue cells into the plasma where it can remain as dissolved CO_2 or hydrate to form hydrogen ion and bicarbonate ion. Because hydrogen ion is buffered by plasma proteins, bicarbonate ion builds up in concentration. This hydration reaction progresses slowly in plasma due to the absence of carbonic anhydrase. Very little CO_2 binds to plasma protein. Consequently, most of the CO_2 diffuses into the red blood cells where it participates in three storage mechanisms: (*1*) dissolved CO_2 in the red cell; (*2*) bound to Hb as carbamino, which is part of the CO_2 Bohr effect that reduces Hb–O_2 affinity; and (*3*) most of the CO_2 in the red cell rapidly undergoes hydration (because of intraerythrocytic carbonic anhydrase) to form H^+ and HCO_3^-. H^+ is buffered by Hb, producing the fixed-acid Bohr effect. The bicarbonate concentration builds up to excessive levels, and some HCO_3^- moves to the plasma via the membrane bicarbonate–chloride exchange transporter. One chloride ion is moved into the red cell in exchange for each bicarbonate ion that moves out of the red cell. This ion

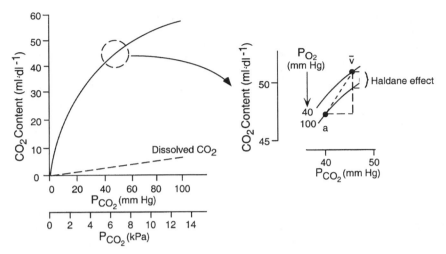

Figure 6.4. Carbon dioxide equilibrium curve. Total CO_2 content is shown as a solid curve. Dissolved CO_2 is shown as a dashed line. The inset shows two total CO_2 content curves for two different P_{O_2} levels demonstrating the Haldane effect.

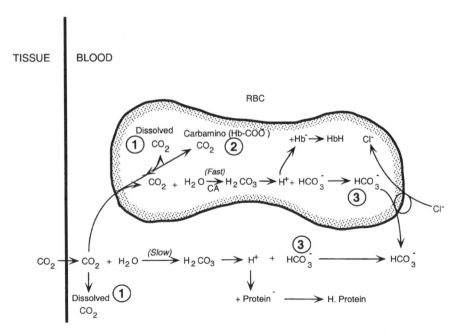

Figure 6.5. Schematic of carbon dioxide transport mechanisms in the blood. Carbonic anhydrase (CA) is contained only within the red blood cell (RBC).

exchange is called the *Hamburger shift*. Because there is an increase in the number of osmotically active ions within the red cells, some water will also diffuse into the cells, causing them to swell. This results in a red cell volume and therefore hematocrit of venous blood greater than those of arterial blood.

CO_2 Equilibrium Curve

The relationship between CO_2 content and P_{CO_2} is curvilinear but is much closer to a straight line than the O_2 equilibrium curve (Fig. 6.4). Over the normal physiological range (35 to 50 mm Hg), the CO_2 equilibrium curve is nearly linear and is treated as if it were straight. The CO_2 content in blood is much higher than the O_2 content, owing to the large bicarbonate storage pool.

The physiological CO_2 equilibrium curve has a steeper slope that results from the Haldane effect (Fig. 6.4, inset). The mixed venous point lies on a CO_2 equilibrium curve appropriate for 75% O_2 saturation. The arterial point lies on another curve (shifted to the right) appropriate for 97% O_2 saturation. During gas exchange, both O_2 and CO_2 are being exchanged at the same time. As CO_2 is lost in the lung and blood moves down the CO_2 equilibrium curve, O_2 uptake by the blood causes the CO_2 equilibrium curve to shift to the right. The vertical distance between the arterial and mixed venous points is equivalent to the total amount of CO_2 exchanged. The distance between the two CO_2 curves represents the CO_2 content exchanged by the Haldane effect. The decrease in CO_2 content, in the absence of a change in the O_2 content, is due to changes in bicarbonate and dissolved CO_2.

Dynamics of Carbon Dioxide Exchange

CO_2 exchange is greatly enhanced by the enzyme carbonic anhydrase (CA). CA is available within the erythrocyte to facilitate the CO_2 hydration reaction, allowing CO_2 to be converted rapidly to bicarbonate. In addition, lung CA is available on the vascular endothelial surface to enhance the rate of conversion within the plasma. If the bicarbonate storage mechanism were not available, the body would require a much greater venous–arterial partial pressure difference in order to transfer the same amount of CO_2. Calculations have shown that blocking lung CA would require a compensatory increase in the venous–arterial P_{CO_2} difference ($\Delta P_{CO_{2v-a}}$) of about 10 mm Hg at rest and 20 mm Hg during exercise. Complete inhibition of both lung and erythrocyte CA would require an increase in $\Delta P_{CO_{2v-a}}$ to about 40 mm Hg at rest and 75 mm Hg at exercise. Thus inhibition of CA can have a significant effect on CO_2 exchange.

In addition, the bicarbonate–chloride exchange process limits the speed of the CO_2 equilibration process within blood because the hydration reaction is increased markedly by carbonic anhydrase. Complete inhibition of erythrocyte anion exchange would require a compensatory increase in cardiac output of 30% to 40%, or an increase in $\Delta P_{CO_{2v-a}}$ from 6 to 8 mm Hg at rest and from 12 to 16 mm Hg during moderate exercise.

Arterial and Venous Carbon Dioxide Content

Carbon dioxide equilibrium occurs between alveolar gas and pulmonary capillary blood. Arterial P_{CO_2} is virtually identical to alveolar P_{CO_2}, which is determined by the balance between alveolar ventilation and CO_2 production (see Chapter 4). Arterial CO_2 content is then determined by arterial P_{CO_2} and the CO_2 equilibrium curve.

Mixed venous ($\bar{v}$) CO_2 content (C) depends on the balance between CO_2 production and cardiac output, as described by the Fick principle (cf Eq. 1.16):

$$C\bar{v}_{CO_2} = Ca_{CO_2} + \frac{\dot{V}_{CO_2}}{\dot{Q}} \tag{6.8}$$

Mixed venous P_{CO_2} is determined by the CO_2 equilibrium curve and $C\bar{v}_{CO_2}$. If $\dot{Q}$ increases or $\dot{V}_{CO_2}$ decreases, both $C\bar{v}_{CO_2}$ and $P\bar{v}_{CO_2}$ will decrease. The opposite occurs with a decrease in $\dot{Q}$ or an increase in $\dot{V}_{CO_2}$.

Oxygen uptake and CO_2 production are linked via metabolism. Under normal circumstances the respiratory quotient (see Chapter 4) is around 0.8:

$$RQ = \frac{\dot{V}_{CO_2}}{\dot{V}_{O_2}} = \frac{\dot{Q}\,(C\bar{v}_{CO_2} - Ca_{CO_2})}{\dot{Q}\,(Ca_{O_2} - C\bar{v}_{O_2})} = 0.8 \tag{6.9}$$

The normal (a–$\bar{v}$) O_2 content difference of 5 ml · dl^{-1} results in a ($\bar{v}$–a) CO_2 content difference of 4.0 (= 0.8 × 5) ml · dl^{-1}. If the balance between $\dot{V}_{O_2}$ and $\dot{Q}$ changes, both $(C\bar{v}_{CO_2} - Ca_{CO_2})$ and $(Ca_{O_2} - C\bar{v}_{O_2})$ will change. The ratio of the two differences will be affected by metabolism in the steady state or by transient changes in blood buffers (see Chapter 7).

Tissue Gas Exchange

Gas exchange processes in the peripheral tissues are essentially opposite from those in the lungs. The anatomical relationships and dynamics are, however, quite different. In the tissues, O_2 is unloaded from the blood and diffuses to the mitochondria, where metabolism converts O_2 to CO_2 and energy. CO_2 must then diffuse to blood for elimination by transport to the lungs. Tissue O_2 delivery must be re-sponsive to the variable demands made by different tissues as well as conditions of stress imposed by the environment, exercise, or disease.

Cellular Metabolism

In all cells, substrates (carbohydrates, proteins, and fats) are utilized to produce energy in the form of adenosine triphosphate (ATP). Cells require this energy in order to survive. The process of oxidative metabolism (also called aerobic metab-olism) uses O_2 and produces CO_2. If O_2 is not present in sufficient quantity, oxi-dative metabolism slows down, and, in the absence of O_2, it stops. Under such circumstances, energy can be produced by glycolysis (also called anaerobic metab-olism). Glycolysis is, however, much less efficient at producing energy (less than one-tenth the amount produced by aerobic metabolism as measured by ATP pro-duction) and produces lactate, a by-product that is more difficult to eliminate than the CO_2 produced by oxidative metabolism.

Mitochondria, the site of oxidation, are distributed around cells and provide energy (Fig. 6.6). Fatty acids, pyruvate, and amino acids are transported through the mitochondrial membrane into the interior of the mitochondria. They are pro-cessed into substances that enter the citrate cycle where reduced nicotinamide ad-enine dinucleotide (NADH) is produced. NADH then diffuses into the cristae, to be oxidized by a respiratory-chain enzyme complex with flavin mononucleotide as a coenzyme. In addition, succinate diffuses into the cristae and releases a hydrogen

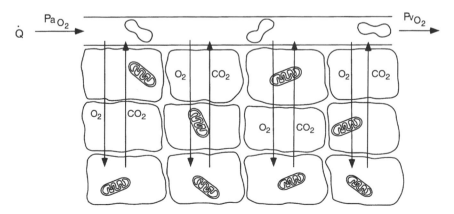

Figure 6.6. Schematic of tissue gas exchange. O_2 diffuses from the capillary to the cells, where it is utilized in the mitochondria. CO_2 diffuses in the opposite direction.

with flavin adenine dinucleotide as a coenzyme. Electrons are transported down the chain, eventually causing O_2 to reduce by combining with free hydrogen ions to form water. The energy from this reaction is used to synthesize ATP.

Distribution of Blood to Cells via Perfusion

In the blood, O_2 is carried to the tissues primarily by Hb, which is contained solely within the erythrocytes. The amount of O_2 carried to a particular tissue depends directly on the amount of perfusion of that tissue as well as the O_2 content of the blood. Any changes in local perfusion can thus have a profound effect on O_2 delivery to the tissue in question. The actual amount of O_2 delivered to any tissue is governed by the Fick principle (see Eq. 6.5), which is based on conservation of mass and states that O_2 delivery to a tissue is equal to tissue perfusion multiplied by the difference between arterial and venous O_2 contents.

Diffusion of Oxygen and Carbon Dioxide

Oxygen is delivered to the tissue capillaries by convection and diffuses through the tissue to the cells and metabolizing mitochondria. These processes are highly dependent on the diffusion distances in the tissue.

Unloading of O_2 by Hb in the red cells is governed by the Hb–O_2 equilibrium curve. Once the O_2 molecule leaves the Hb, its movement is governed by passive diffusion. The partial pressure difference of O_2 determines the rate at which O_2 diffuses between two points. Figure 6.6 is a schematic representation of tissue with a capillary and surrounding cells through which both O_2 and CO_2 diffuse. The cells are distributed in three dimensions around the capillary. Oxygen diffuses in all directions from the location where it is released from Hb. The major direction of diffusion is, however, likely to occur in a radial direction perpendicular to the capillary.

The O_2 partial pressure in the tissue decreases as the distance from the capillary increases and from the arterial end to the venous end of the capillary. Computer models have been used to calculate the O_2 partial pressure at various positions within tissue. Figure 6.7 shows such a calculation for a tissue composed of adjacent cylinders of cells fed by single, parallel capillaries. This classic *Krogh cylinder* demonstrates that P_{O_2} decreases radically until a point is reached half way between the two identical, parallel, cocurrent capillaries. In addition, at any radial distance from the capillary, the P_{O_2} reduces as the axial distance along the capillary increases. The actual contour of P_{O_2} in any particular tissue depends on the orientation of capillaries in the tissue, the relative perfusion through each capillary and the distribution of mitochondria through the tissue.

Carbon dioxide partial pressure is distributed in a similar pattern, but, because

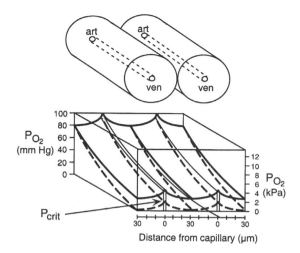

Figure 6.7. Calculated P_{O_2} profile in tissue surrounding a capillary. Profiles are shown for a classic Krogh cylinder in the normal state (solid lines) and low-flow state (dashed lines). P_{crit} is the critical venous P_{O_2} below which the O_2 partial pressure is insufficient to provide enough O_2 to the mitochondria most distal from the venous end of the capillary. (Adapted from Schmidt RF, Thews G. *Human Physiology*. New York: Springer-Verlag, 1983, p 514.)

CO_2 is produced at the mitochondria and taken up by the blood, the diffusion gradients are reversed: P_{CO_2} is highest in the cells and lowest at the arterial end of the capillary. Because CO_2 has a much higher solubility than O_2, P_{CO_2} would be expected to have a smaller range than P_{O_2}. In average tissue, blood P_{CO_2} ranges from 40 mm Hg at the arterial end to 46 mm Hg at the venous end.

The tissue exchanges of O_2 and CO_2 are linked by virtue of their interaction in the Hb molecule. The uptake of CO_2 as blood is passing through the capillary and the Bohr effect shift the O_2 equilibrium curve to the right, releases oxygen at a higher P_{O_2}, enhancing the diffusion partial pressure difference between the blood and the mitochondria and increasing diffusion. In a similar manner, release of O_2 and the Haldane effect cause the CO_2 equilibrium curve to shift to the left and allows CO_2 uptake at a lower P_{CO_2}. This enhances the diffusion partial pressure difference between the mitochondria and the blood, as well as diffusion. This Bohr-Haldane interaction is much more important for facilitating CO_2 exchange ($\sim 40\%$) than for O_2 exchange ($\sim 2\%$).

Partial Pressure of Oxygen Distribution in Tissue

As shown by the calculations in Figure 6.7, P_{O_2} varies at different points in tissue. The highest P_{O_2} is near the arterial end of the capillary, while the lowest P_{O_2} is in the regions most distant from the venous end of the capillary. Fortunately, the mitochondria metabolize at a constant rate until P_{O_2} is reduced to 1 mm Hg or less.

The mitochondria most likely to be affected by limitations in O_2 delivery are most radially distant from the venous end of the capillary. For example, reduced

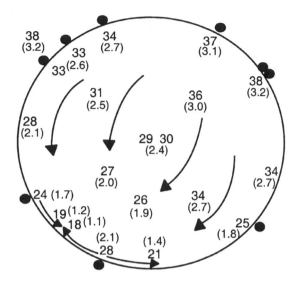

Figure 6.8. P_{O_2} distribution measured in a muscle cell during severe exercise. Solid circles represent capillaries. Myoglobin saturation is indicated with P_{O_2} in parentheses. Arrows show direction of oxygen flux. (Adapted from Honig CR, Gayeski TEJ, Groebe K. Myoglobin and oxygen gradients. In: Crystal RG, West JB, editors. *The Lung: Scientific Foundations.* New York: Raven Press, 1991, pp 1489–1496.)

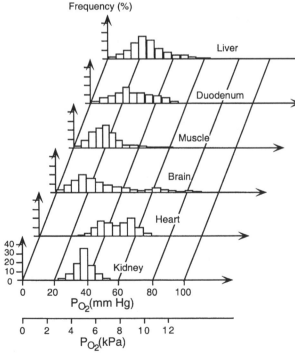

Figure 6.9. P_{O_2} histograms obtained from different organs. (Adapted from Kessler M, Höper J, Pohl U. Monitoring of local P_{O_2} in skeletal muscle of critically ill patients. In: Berk JL, editor. *Handbook of Critical Care,* 2nd ed. Boston: Little, Brown & Co, 1982, pp 599–609.)

perfusion with the same tissue O_2 consumption will increase extraction of O_2 and will lower the venous P_{O_2} and the P_{O_2} in the cells most distant from the venous end. Likewise, an increase in O_2 consumption and unchanged perfusion will lower venous P_{O_2} and further reduce P_{O_2} in distant cells. The critical P_{O_2} is the venous P_{O_2} at which tissue O_2 delivery begins to be limited.

The theoretical profile of P_{O_2} in tissue is likely to be perturbed by local anisotropies of diffusion resistance. Measurements in muscle cells show very small changes in P_{O_2} throughout the cell (Fig. 6.8), indicating that diffusion resistance across the cell membrane is much greater than within the cell.

The distribution of P_{O_2} within the tissue has been measured with small glass microelectrodes. Figure 6.9 shows P_{O_2} distributions in different types of tissue. Each tissue has a different distribution. In the gray matter of the brain cortex, the range is very wide. Most tissues have a P_{O_2} between 10 and 40 mm Hg, although P_{O_2} values in some regions of tissue are lower than 10 mm Hg or higher than 40 mm Hg. It is likely that distribution of blood flow, diffusion properties, and/or oxygen uptake may vary in each of these tissues.

Interactions Between Components of Oxygen Transport

Several variables affect O_2 delivery to a particular tissue, including ventilation, Hb concentration, cardiac output, and tissue microvascular flow pattern. Different tissues utilize a different balance of variables to provide O_2 delivery under different conditions. Figure 6.10 shows the relationships among these variables as they influence O_2 delivery. For a particular organ or tissue, the area of the hatched rectangle corresponds to O_2 consumption, calculated using the Fick principle as the product of blood flow and the arteriovenous O_2 content difference (see Eq. 6.5). When $\dot{V}_{O_2}$ is limited, any of the reserves may be tapped to meet additional O_2 demand and maintain $\dot{V}_{O_2}$.

In response to high altitude exposure, the body increases Hb concentration (erythropoietic reserve), and this increases arterial O_2 content. Another response to moderate altitude exposure is an increase in P_{50} (O_2 equilibrium curve reserve), which increases venous P_{O_2} and enhances the ability of O_2 to diffuse to the cells most distant from the venous end of the capillary. Exposure to high altitude also increases the number of capillaries (microcirculatory and tissue reserve), which reduces the diffusion distances. At altitudes above sea level, hyperventilation increases alveolar P_{O_2} and arterial O_2 content (ventilatory reserve—this mechanism is not useful at sea level because of the relative flatness of the O_2 equilibrium curve for $P_{O_2} > 100$ mm Hg). Adaptation to altitude causes a growth of additional tissue capillaries (microcirculatory and tissue reserve), which reduces the distance for O_2 diffusion from capillaries. Any compensation allowing greater extraction of O_2 from

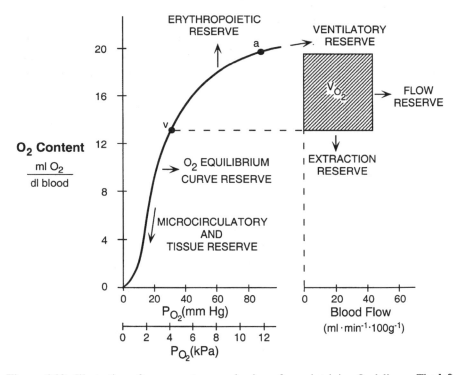

Figure 6.10. Illustration of compensatory mechanisms for maintaining O_2 delivery. The **left graph** is a standard O_2 equilibrium curve. The **right graph** is an O_2 content versus blood flow curve, with the cross-hatched area representing O_2 consumption. (Adapted from Woodson RD. O_2 transport: DPG and P_{50}. *Basics of Respiratory Disease*, vol 5. New York: American Thoracic Society, 1977, pp 1–6.

blood (extraction reserve) enhances O_2 delivery with a given tissue blood flow. Increasing blood flow to tissue (flow reserve) also enhances O_2 delivery.

Further Reading

1. Baumann R, Bartels H, Bauer C. Blood oxygen transport. In: Farhi LE, Tenney SM, editors. *Handbook of Physiology*, Section 3, *The Respiratory System*, vol IV, *Gas Exchange*. Bethesda, MD: American Physiological Society, 1987, pp 147–172.
2. Coburn RF, Forman HJ. Carbon monoxide toxicity. In: Farhi LE, Tenney SM, editors. *Handbook of Physiology*, Section 3, *The Respiratory System*, vol IV, *Gas Exchange*. Bethesda, MD: American Physiological Society, 1987, pp 147–172.
3. Klocke RE. Carbon dioxide transort. In: Crystal RG, West, JB, Weibel ER, Barns PJ,

editors. *The Lung: Scientific Foundations*, 2nd ed, vol 2. Philadelphia: Lippincott-Raven, 1997, pp 1633–1642.

4. Wagner PD, Hoppeler H. Saltin B. Determinants of maximal oxygen uptake. In: Crystal RG, West JB, Weibel ER, Barns PJ, *The Lung: Scientific Foundations*, 2nd ed, vol. 2. Philadelphia: Lippincott-Raven, 1997, pp 2033–2041.

5. Woodson RD. O_2 transport: DPG and P_{50}. *Basics of Respiratory Disease*, vol 5. New York: American Thoracic Society, 1977, pp 1–6.

Study Questions

6.1 Describe quantitatively how normal arterial O_2 content and saturation change if Hb concentration is reduced to 80% of normal in an individual with normal alveolar P_{O_2}.

6.2. What factors affect Hb–O_2 affinity?

6.3. Describe the CO_2 storage mechanisms in blood.

6.4. Compare the relative importance of the Bohr effect on O_2 exchange to that of the Haldane effect on CO_2 exchange.

6.5. How can the Fick principle for O_2 exchange be used to measure cardiac output?

6.6. Is aerobic or anaerobic metabolism the most efficient for energy production?

6.7. Discuss the manner by which O_2 and CO_2 interaction with Hb enhances the exchange of both O_2 and CO_2 in tissue.

6.8. Describe how the tissue P_{O_2} distribution would change with an increase in tissue perfusion and no other changes. What would the change be with only a decrease in hematocrit?

6.9. Discuss the compensatory mechanisms available to normalize tissue O_2 delivery during times of stress.

7

Pulmonary Gas Exchange

Ventilation delivers O_2 to and removes CO_2 from the lung. The circulation transports O_2 and CO_2 between the lung and the peripheral tissue. The mechanisms for the exchange of O_2 and CO_2 between the alveolar gas and pulmonary capillary blood are the subject of this chapter. These passive mechanisms can be influenced by outside factors, such as gravity and barometric pressure, and they are altered by most respiratory diseases. The factors determining efficiency of the exchange process can be separated into two major components: diffusion and matching of ventilation to perfusion ($\dot{V}_A/\dot{Q}$). Furthermore, diffusion can be divided into three components: the gas phase, the alveolocapillary membrane, and the blood. The $\dot{V}_A/\dot{Q}$ ratio spans a broad range from zero (shunt, no ventilation) to infinity (dead space, no perfusion). Shunt is discussed as a special entity, although it represents only the extreme lower limit of the $\dot{V}_A/\dot{Q}$ range.

Diffusion

Diffusive flux through a barrier separating two regions of differing gas partial pressures is governed by Fick's first law of diffusion* (already derived in Chapter 1):

$$\dot{V} = \frac{-\beta_m \mathscr{D} A}{\ell} (P_1 - P_2) \tag{7.1}$$

While moving between alveolar gas and capillary blood, each gas species is subject to the same anatomically related limitations (A, ℓ). Each gas, however, has

---

*Here the gas flow is considered as a volume flow ($\dot{V}$) rather than a mass or molar flow ($\dot{M}$) indicated in Figure 1.6.

a different solubility (β_m) and diffusivity ($\mathscr{D}$) in the membrane (m) barrier. All anatomical and gas-related parameters in equation 7.1 are generally lumped together under the term *diffusing capacity of the lung* (D_L) and expressed as a simplification of equation 7.1:

$$\dot{V} = D_L \, (P_A - P_b) \tag{7.2}$$

D_L represents the conductance for diffusion between the alveolar space partial pressure, P_A, and the blood partial pressure, P_b.

Gas molecules diffuse relatively rapidly within the alveolar gas due to the long distances traveled between collisions. It is generally assumed that the effective diffusion conductance in alveolar gas is very large so that it is a negligible component of the overall resistance to gas diffusion between alveolar gas and blood.

Diffusive resistance across the alveolocapillary membrane (composed of the surfactant lining layer, alveolar epithelium, interstitial space, and capillary endothelium) is much more important. Fick's first law of diffusion (Eq. 7.1) enables us to estimate the ratio of lung diffusing capacities for O_2 and for CO_2. CO_2 has a solubility in water (the primary component of the alveolocapillary membrane) 24 times that of O_2 and a molecular weight of 44 compared with 32 for O_2. Therefore, the relative diffusing capacities are

$$\frac{D_{CO_2}}{D_{O_2}} = \frac{\beta m_{CO_2}}{\beta m_{O_2}} \times \frac{\mathscr{D}_{CO_2}}{\mathscr{D}_{O_2}} = 24 \, \frac{\dfrac{1}{\sqrt{44}}}{\dfrac{1}{\sqrt{32}}} \cong 20 \tag{7.3}$$

From this it is apparent that CO_2 diffuses about 20 times faster than O_2 through the alveolocapillary membrane. This estimate, of course, depends on the validity of the assumption of water-like behavior of the alveolocapillary membrane. This estimation applies only to the membrane portion of diffusing capacity and not to the chemical reaction term (see below).

From our knowledge of anatomy and of Fick's diffusion relationships, the dynamics of gas exchange as blood passes through the pulmonary capillary can be calculated. Because of present technical limitations, it is impossible to measure directly the O_2 and CO_2 exchange across the alveolocapillary membrane. Theoretical predictions indicate that the relative equilibration of gas with blood (b) at any point X along the length (X_0) of a pulmonary capillary depends on the balance between diffusing capacity ($D = \beta_m \mathscr{D} A/\ell$ from Eqs. 7.1 and 7.2) and perfusion, as described by the ratio $D/\dot{Q}\beta_b$ (see Fig. 7.1):

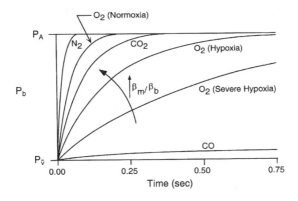

Figure 7.1. Equilibration profiles for various gases in pulmonary capillary blood. Gas partial pressure is plotted against time along the capillary. Curves for gases with differing $D/\dot{Q}\,\beta_b$ are shown; recall that $D/\dot{Q}\beta_b = \mathcal{D}A\beta_m/\beta_b\,\dot{Q}\ell$. (Adapted from Piiper J, Scheid P. Blood-gas equilibration in lungs. In: West JB, editor. *Pulmonary Gas Exchange,* vol 1. New York: Academic Press, 1980, pp 131–171.)

$$\frac{P_b - P_v}{P_A - P_v} = 1 - e^{-\Phi} \qquad (7.4)$$

where $\Phi = (D/\dot{Q}\beta_b)(X/X_0) = (\mathcal{D}A/\ell)(\beta_m/\beta_b)(1/\dot{Q})(X/X_0)$.

For the respiratory gases (O_2 and CO_2) with nonlinear blood equilibrium curves, β_b is an effective solubility between the arterial and venous points ($\beta_b = [C_a - C_v]/[P_a - P_v]$). An increased diffusing capacity or decreased perfusion will cause a more rapid equilibration of blood with alveolar gas. Because the diffusing capacity, D, includes a term for the solubility of gas in the alveolocapillary membrane (β_m), the ratio $D/\dot{Q}\beta_b$ ($=\mathcal{D}A\beta_m/\beta_b\dot{Q}\ell$) dependents on the ratio of the solubility of the gas in the membrane (β_m) to that in blood (β_b). At the extreme, when $\Phi = 0$, there is no alveolar gas exchange, and $P_b = P_v$. When Φ is large, the gas equilibrates easily within the transit time, and $P_b = P_A$. For inert gases (those that do not react chemically in the blood), β_m is approximately equal to β_b, and therefore Φ is large. For O_2, $\beta_m/\beta_b \ll 1$ because there is no hemoglobin in the tissue barrier. Therefore, $D/\dot{Q}\beta_b$ for O_2 is much smaller than $D/\dot{Q}\beta_b$ for an inert gas. Inert gas equilibrates very rapidly, usually within one-tenth of the pulmonary capillary transit time. Oxygen takes longer to equilibrate, and in the hypoxic situation β_b is reduced and O_2 may not equilibrate between alveolar gas and end-capillary blood.

No additional net exchange of gas occurs after equilibrium is reached. The amount of gas exchanged per minute depends on the difference between equilibrium content of the blood and the incoming venous content of blood times the amount of blood flow per minute. Gas exchange with a high $D/\dot{Q}\beta_b$ is directly dependent on blood flow and is said to be perfusion limited. Oxygen binds to hemoglobin, and thus the $\beta_m/\beta_b \ll 1$ and $D/\dot{Q}\beta_b$ turn out to be about 10 during normoxic breathing. This means that O_2 will equilibrate within one-third of the capillary transit time and is therefore perfusion limited. In hypoxia, blood is de-saturated for longer periods during pulmonary capillary transit, and the effective blood solubility (β_b, the slope of the line $[\Delta C/\Delta P = (C_a - C_v/(P_a - P_v)]$ connecting the arterial and venous points in Fig. 6.1) is increased even more than during normoxia, causing a lower $D/\dot{Q}\beta_b$ and a longer equilibration time. As long as equilibrium is reached with $P_{A_{O_2}}$, the amount of O_2 exchanged depends on perfusion. Lowering alveolar P_{O_2} below 40 mm Hg will result in pulmonary end-capillary to alveolar disequilibrium, even when lung diffusing capacity and cardiac output are normal. In this case, O_2 exchange is both perfusion and diffusion limited. Carbon monoxide, another gas of physiological interest, has a much higher β_b than O_2 because of its high affinity for hemoglobin (250 times the O_2 affinity). CO has a $D/\dot{Q}\beta_b$ on the order of 0.03, making it extremely slow to equilibrate. This gas is diffusion limited in the lung and well suited for measuring the diffusion properties of the lung.

Another major resistance to O_2 exchange lies within the red cell. The resistance of the red cell includes the diffusion through a densely packed hemoglobin solution, which includes resistance related to the chemical reaction of O_2 with hemoglobin in blood. The membrane and red cell resistances are arranged in series. Any ex-changing gas species (X) must move through both resistances. Because the pressure drop across the entire resistance is the sum of the pressure drops across each re-sistance in series,

$$\frac{P_A - P_{Hb}}{\dot{V}_X} = \frac{P_A - P_p}{\dot{V}_X} + \frac{P_p - P_{Hb}}{\dot{V}_X} \tag{7.5}$$

where P_A, P_p, and P_{Hb} are partial pressures in alveolar gas and plasma and the equivalent partial pressure of O_2 bound to hemoglobin, respectively. Rearrangement of equation 7.2 with substitution into equation 7.5 gives the following relationships:

$$\frac{1}{D_L} = \frac{1}{D_M} + \frac{1}{\Theta V_c} \tag{7.6}$$

Each of the terms in equations 7.5 and 7.6 are resistances, and these equations simply state that the overall resistance is the sum of the two resistances in series. Thus, the inverse of the total lung diffusing capacity (D_L) is equal to the sum of the inverse of the membrane diffusing capacity (D_M) and the inverse of the red cell diffusing capacity (made up of V_c, the capillary volume, and Θ, a chemical reaction term). For O_2, each component represents about half of the total resistance. For

CO_2, the red cell component is much greater than the membrane component because the multiple chemical reactions and diffusive resistances are involved in blood CO_2 storage (see Chapter 6).

Measurement of Lung Diffusing Capacity

Carbon monoxide exchange, which is independent of perfusion, can be used to measure the lung diffusing capacity. Because of the high affinity of hemoglobin for CO, the P_{CO} in blood remains nearly zero ($P_{bco} \approx 0$) throughout the entire capillary transit. Thus the Fick equation for CO becomes

$$\dot{V}_{CO} = D_{LCO} (P_{ACO} - P_{bco}) = D_{LCO} P_{ACO} \qquad (7.7)$$

Because the uptake of CO is directly dependent on P_{ACO}, the P_{ACO} exhibits an exponential decrease with time during a breath-hold.

To measure the single breath diffusing capacity, the subject inspires a vital capacity of gas containing 0.35% CO, 5% He, 21% O_2, and the rest N_2. After 10 seconds of breath-holding, the subject exhales, and an end-exhalation gas sample is collected. Because the uptake is exponential at a rate dependent on diffusing capacity, exhaled P_{CO} is compared with the initial P_{CO} to calculate D_{LCO}. Helium (or some other poorly soluble gas) is used as an indicator of lung volume (by dilution) allowing calculation of initial P_{ACO}. An alternate approach for measuring D_{LCO} is the steady-state diffusing capacity, which is measured while the subject breathes CO (0.1%) for a period of several minutes. CO uptake is determined by using the open circuit technique (described in Chapter 4), and alveolar P_{CO} is estimated by determining the physiological dead space by evaluating CO_2 exchange efficiency. Once the diffusing capacity for CO is known, the diffusing capacity for O_2 can be estimated from the gas physical properties by using a relationship similar to that in equation 7.3. The D_{LCO} is often used as an index to evaluate the pulmonary gas exchange efficiency in patients with lung disease. The primary mechanism for a reduction of D_{LCO} in lung disease is the increased heterogeneity of ventilation—not a thickening of the alveolocapillary barrier.

Oxygen and Carbon Dioxide Equilibration

The rate of equilibration of O_2 and CO_2 in blood while passing through the pulmonary capillary can be calculated with equation 7.4. A complication is the nonlinearity of the O_2 and CO_2 equilibrium curves. The calculated profile for O_2 shows that equilibrium is achieved when the blood reaches about one-third of the capillary length (Fig. 7.2). If the diffusing capacity is decreased by disease, the blood must travel farther along the capillary before equilibrium is reached. At sea level the

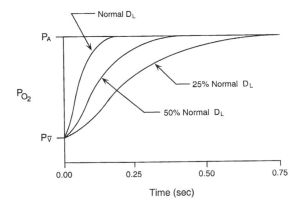

Figure 7.2. Equilibration of O_2 in pulmonary capillary blood. Profiles are shown for normal and reduced lung diffusing capacity. A time of 0.75 second corresponds to approximately one capillary transit time.

diffusing capacity must be reduced to less than 25% of normal before arterial deoxygenation occurs. At high altitude, because of reductions of inspired P_{O_2}, arterial P_{O_2}, and mixed venous P_{O_2} and an increased effective blood O_2 solubility, the equilibration is slower and deoxygenation is even more likely (see Chapter 11). Exercise also increases the likelihood of deoxygenation because increased cardiac output reduces the pulmonary capillary transit time (see Chapter 12).

Carbon dioxide equilibrium calculations are more uncertain because of the many reactions involved in CO_2 carriage. Calculations show that equilibrium occurs within one-half of the normal capillary transit time (Fig. 7.3). Decreased CO_2 membrane diffusing capacity (Dm_{CO_2}) has very little effect on CO_2 equilibrium because the membrane component represents only a small fraction of the total lung CO_2 diffusion resistance as most of the resistance for CO_2 is in the red cell.

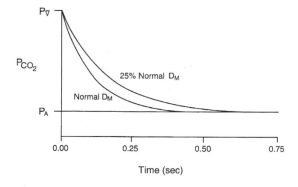

Figure 7.3. Equilibration of CO_2 in pulmonary capillary blood. Profiles are shown for normal and reduced membrane diffusing capacity (D_m).

Shunt

Shunt is the passage of deoxygenated blood from the venous circulation to the arterial side of the circulation without picking up O_2. The relative deoxygenation of arterial blood depends to a large degree on the magnitude of the shunt. Potential sources of shunted blood are many. The thebesian circulation perfuses the left ventricle myocardium and empties deoxygenated blood directly into the left ventricle. Some of the deoxygenated blood coming from the bronchial circulation empties into the pulmonary veins, which also contributes deoxygenated blood to the arterial circulation. A major source of shunt can be perfusion of atelectatic alveoli (alveoli that are collapsed and not ventilated). In some individuals, congenital defects can result in right-to-left shunt through atrial or ventricular septal defects or transposition of the great arteries. In some species, such as lizards, large right-to-left (and left-to-right) shunts across the incomplete ventricular septum exist normally. Right-to-left shunt contributes to arterial deoxygenation, but left-to-right shunt does not.

An example of a lung with a normal region and a shunt (or shunts) region is shown in Figure 7.4. In this case, 50% of the cardiac output goes through each region, resulting in a 50% shunt. To determine the O_2 content of the mixed arterial blood, we must apply the principle of conservation of mass in order to determine a total (t) number of O_2 molecules coming to the mixing point and thus determine the number of O_2 molecules leaving the mixing point (see Fig. 7.4):

$$\dot{Q}_s \, C\bar{v}_{O_2} + (\dot{Q}_t - \dot{Q}_s) \, Cc_{O_2} = \dot{Q}_t \, Ca_{O_2} \tag{7.8}$$

where C_c is end-capillary content.

Algebraic manipulation of equation 7.8 yields the *Berggren shunt equation*:

$$\frac{\dot{Q}_s}{\dot{Q}_t} = \frac{Cc_{O_2} - Ca_{O_2}}{Cc_{O_2} - C\bar{v}_{O_2}} \tag{7.9}$$

If the inspired O_2 fraction is 1.0, alveolar P_{O2} is very high in all ventilated alveoli, the end-capillary O_2 content is similar, and $\dot{V}_A/\dot{Q}$ heterogeneity will have very little influence on the difference between alveolar and arterial gas (see below). When $FI_{O_2} = 1.0$, the shunt fraction can be determined directly from arterial O_2 content, end-capillary O_2 content (calculated from alveolar P_{O_2}), and mixed venous O_2 content. If equation 7.9 is applied to someone breathing less than 100% O_2, the resulting determination of shunt is called the *venous admixture*. Venous admix-

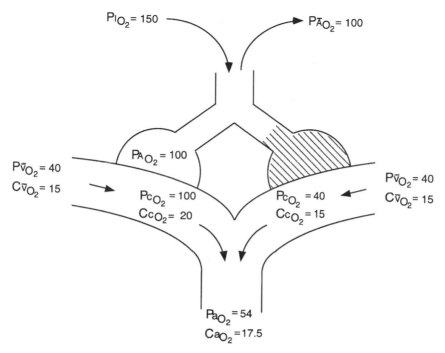

Figure 7.4. Two-compartment lung with 50% of perfusion to one normal alveolus and 50% to shunt. P_{O_2} values are shown in mm Hg. O_2 content values are in volumes percent (ml · dl^{-1}). Shaded area represents a fluid-filled alveolus. When determining the mixed O_2 content and partial pressure, consider only the weighted content and not the weighted partial pressure. (Adapted from B. Culver, Ed., Human Biology 541 syllabus: *The Respiratory System.* University of Washington, Seattle: ASUW Publishing.)

ture consists of pure shunt plus a component due to $\dot{V}_A/\dot{Q}$ heterogeneity (alveolar dead space).

Administration of 100% O_2 to a lung with 50% shunt will increase the arterial P_{O_2} only slightly (Fig. 7.5). No additional O_2 is added to shunted blood. Because hemoglobin approaches saturation at a P_{O_2} of 100 mm Hg, increasing P_{O_2} to 673 mm Hg in the normal alveolus increases O_2 content only slightly (to 22 ml · dl^{-1}), primarily via an increase in dissolved O_2 content. The slightly increased mixed arterial O_2 content (18.5 ml · dl^{-1}) causes a slightly increased partial pressure due to the steepness of the O_2 equilibrium curve at that point. In the presence of large shunts, increasing inspired O_2 concentration has little effect on arterial P_{O_2}. Increasing inspired P_{O_2} as a means of increasing arterial P_{O_2} however, becomes more effective as shunt percentage decreases. Increased O_2 fraction for prolonged periods

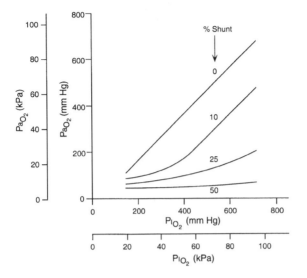

Figure 7.5. An increase occurs in arterial P_{O_2} as inspired P_{O_2} is increased. Curves are shown for lungs with varying shunt fractions.

of time may cause other problems: (*1*) oxygen toxicity (increasing lung pathology), (*2*) absorption atelectasis (collapse of the alveolus due to gas absorption by the blood, causing increased shunt), and (*3*) decreased hypoxic pulmonary vasoconstriction (increasing perfusion to hypoxic regions).

A common clinical approach for estimating pulmonary shunt is to administer 100% O_2, measure arterial blood gases, and calculate the alveolar–arterial P_{O_2} difference ($[(A - a] P_{O_2})$ (see Chapter 4). From Figure 7.6, it can be seen that, under conditions of 100% O_2 breathing ($P_{I_{O_2}}$ = 713 mm Hg), the drop in $P_{A_{O_2}}$ is linearly related to shunt up to shunt values of about 25%. This is because of the linear shape of the O_2 equilibrium curve for $P_{O_2} > 150$ mm Hg. The general rule of thumb is that every 1% shunt causes a 20 mm Hg increase in $(A - a)P_{O_2}$. Under normal circumstances of a 5% shunt, the lungs have an $(A - a)P_{O_2}$ of 100 mm Hg. This relationship is true if the following three conditions are present: (*1*) breathing 100% O_2, (*2*) $Pa_{O_2} > 150$ mm Hg (on the linear portion of the O_2 equilibrium curve), and (*3*) normal cardiac output (indicating a normal $Ca_{O_2} - Cv_{O_2}$).

Ventilation/Perfusion Heterogeneity

Every minute, the normal human lung is ventilated with gas and perfused with blood in nearly equal flow rates. If ventilation and perfusion are equally matched throughout the lung, then arterial P_{O_2} and P_{CO_2} will be identical to mixed alveolar

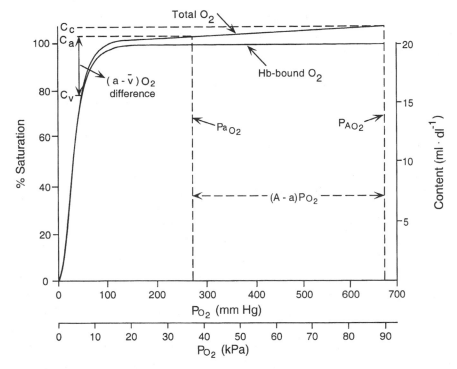

Figure 7.6. Oxygen equilibrium curve demonstrating the effect of shunt while 100% O_2 is breathed. Normally, each 1% shunt corresponds to an $(A - a)P_{O_2}$ of 20 mm Hg. This example shows a 20% shunt resulting in an $(A - a)P_{O_2}$ of 400 mm Hg. (Adapted from B. Culver, Ed., Human Biology 541 syllabus: *The Respiratory System.* University of Washington, Seattle: ASUW Publishing.)

P_{O_2} and P_{CO_2}. Several important normal factors (see Chapters 4 and 5), however, cause ventilation and perfusion to be distributed unequally.

In a single alveolus with a constant ventilation and perfusion, the uptake of O_2 is governed by the conservation of mass principle:

$$\dot{V}_{O_2} = \dot{V}_A \, (FI_{O_2} - FA_{O_2}) \tag{7.10}$$

Uptake of oxygen by the blood is governed by the Fick principle:

$$\dot{V}_{O_2} = \dot{Q} \, (Ca_{O_2} - C\bar{v}_{O_2}) \tag{7.11}$$

Consider the dynamic changes that would occur if perfusion were abruptly increased. Because $C\bar{v}_{O_2}$ would not change initially, more O_2 would be taken up by the blood. A greater O_2 uptake for a given ventilation would reduce alveolar P_{O_2}. If alveolar P_{O_2} decreases, then end-capillary P_{O_2} and end-capillary O_2 contents would also decrease. A decrease in arterial content (with a constant $C\bar{v}_{O_2}$) would then decrease O_2 uptake. Eventually, a steady state would be reached with a decrease in both Pa_{O_2} and mean $\dot{V}_A/\dot{Q}$ of the unit. The opposite would occur (an increase in Pa_{O_2}) if perfusion were decreased or ventilation were increased—either condition raising the $\dot{V}_A/\dot{Q}$ ratio in such an alveolus. Thus the P_{O_2} of blood and gas leaving an alveolus depends on the relative ventilation and perfusion of that alveolus.

A two-compartment lung demonstrating the alveolar gas and blood P_{O_2} values is shown in Figure 7.7. The left alveolus has normal ventilation and perfusion and hence a normal P_{O_2} of 100 mm Hg. The right alveolus has an airway constriction and low ventilation. This low $\dot{V}_A/\dot{Q}$ unit has a lower P_{O_2} in both the alveolar gas and end-capillary blood because the delivery of O_2 to the alveolus by the lower ventilation is unable to keep up with the O_2 taken up by the blood. The arterial O_2 content consists of a mixture of the end-capillary O_2 content from each alveolus in proportion to the relative perfusion of each alveolus. In this example, the equal flows produce a mixed arterial O_2 content of 18.5 ml · dl^{-1}, which is halfway between the individual O_2 contents of 20 ml · dl^{-1} and 17 ml · dl^{-1}. The arterial P_{O_2} is then determined by the O_2 content and the O_2 equilibrium curve to be 64 mm Hg. Mixed alveolar P_{O_2} is determined by the relative exhaled ventilation from the two alveoli. In this example, the normal alveolus has twice the ventilation as the low $\dot{V}_A/\dot{Q}$ alveolus, as evidenced by the relative differences between P_{IO_2} and

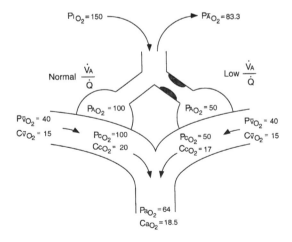

Figure 7.7. A two-compartment lung with 50% of perfusion to one normal alveolus and 50% of perfusion to a low $\dot{V}_A/\dot{Q}$ alveolus. Inspired air has a P_{O_2} of 150 mm Hg. P_{O_2} values are shown in mm Hg. O_2 content values are in ml · dl^{-1}. Shaded areas represent airway narrowing. Assume R = 0.80, F_{IO_2} = 0.21. (Adapted from B. Culver, Ed., Human Biology 541 syllabus: *The Respiratory System*. University of Washington, Seattle: ASUW Publishing.)

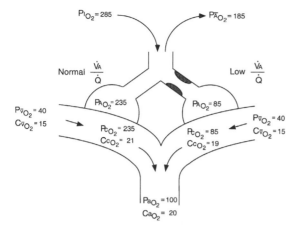

Figure 7.8. A two-compartment lung with 50% of perfusion to one normal alveolus and 50% to a low $\dot{V}_A/\dot{Q}$ alveolus. Inspired gas has a P_{O_2} of 285 mm Hg. P_{O_2} values are shown in mm Hg. O_2 content values are in ml · dl^{-1}. Shaded areas represent airway narrowing. Assume R = 0.80, $F_{I_{O_2}}$ = 0.4. (Adapted from B. Culver, Ed., Human Biology 541 syllabus: *The Respiratory System.* University of Washington, Seattle: ASUW Publishing.)

PA_{O_2} (150 − 100 and 150 − 50, respectively). The ventilation-weighted PA_{O_2} will be 83.3 mm Hg [= (2 × 100 + 1 × 50)/3].

For a patient with $\dot{V}_A/\dot{Q}$ heterogeneity such as that shown in Figure 7.7, it is possible to increase the arterial P_{O_2} by administering gas with increased P_{O_2}. Figure 7.8 shows the same alveoli as in Figure 7.7, with inspired P_{O_2} increased to 285 mm Hg. The normal alveolus P_{O_2} is increased to 235 mm Hg, and the low $\dot{V}_A/\dot{Q}$ alveolus P_{O_2} is increased to 85 mm Hg with a resulting mixed arterial P_{O_2} of 100 mm Hg and mixed alveolar P_{O_2} of 185 mm Hg. Delivery of increased inspired P_{O_2} can help to increase arterial P_{O_2} in a patient with $\dot{V}_A/\dot{Q}$ heterogeneity, but helps to a lesser degree in a patient with hypoxemia due to shunt (see Figs. 7.4 and 7.5), as additional O_2 cannot be added to the shunted blood.

A common approach to describing the influence of $\dot{V}_A/\dot{Q}$ distribution on the exchange of O_2 and CO_2 between alveolar gas and arterial blood is illustrated with the O_2–CO_2 diagram (Fig. 7.9). This diagram describes all alveoli that can exist in a lung with a given mixed venous and inspired gas P_{O_2} and P_{CO_2}. It is constructed as the intersection of lines describing gas exchange from both blood and inspired gas with identical gas exchange ratios (gas R = blood R) and assumed diffusion equilibration between the alveolar gas and end-capillary blood (P_{CO_2} = PA_{O_2} and Pc_{CO_2} = PA_{CO_2}). A three-compartment lung with a severe $\dot{V}_A/\dot{Q}$ heterogeneity is shown. Perfusion is evenly divided between a normal alveolus having a P_{O_2} of 100 mm Hg and a P_{CO_2} of 40 mm Hg and a collapsed alveolus ($\dot{V}_A/\dot{Q}$ = 0) having the equivalent of mixed venous blood with P_{O_2} of 40 mm Hg and P_{CO_2} of 46 mm Hg. Ventilation is evenly divided between the normal alveolus and an alveolus with no

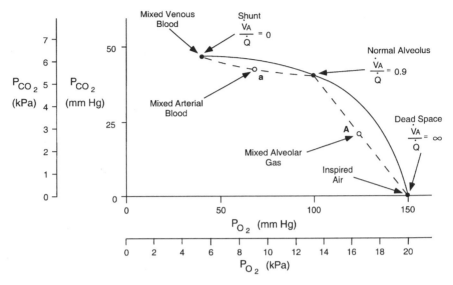

Figure 7.9. O_2–CO_2 diagram. A three-compartment lung is illustrated with the perfusion divided equally between shunt and the normal alveolus. Ventilation is divided equally between dead space and the normal alveolus. Mixed arterial (a) and mixed alveolar (A) points are shown. (Adapted from Rahn H. A concept of mean alveolar air and the ventilation–blood flow relationships during pulmonary gas exchange. *Am J Physiol* 158:21–30, 1949; and Riley RL, Cournand A. 'Ideal' alveolar air and the analysis of ventilation–perfusion relationships in the lungs. *J Appl Physiol* 1:825–847, 1949.)

blood flow ($\dot{V}_A/\dot{Q} = \infty$) having an alveolar gas equivalent to inspired gas; P_{O_2} of 150 mm Hg; and P_{CO_2} of 0 mm Hg. The lung has alveoli spanning the range of $\dot{V}_A/\dot{Q}$ from zero to infinity. Note that low $\dot{V}_A/\dot{Q}$ regions make a marked contribution to the (A − a) P_{O_2} but very little contribution to the (a − A)P_{CO_2}, whereas high $\dot{V}_A/\dot{Q}$ regions contribute to both.

The mixed alveolar gas is a ventilation-weighted average of the gases coming from each alveolus. Because no ventilation comes from the $\dot{V}_A/\dot{Q} = 0$ alveolus, the mixed alveolar point must fall on a line connecting the normal alveolus point to the dead space alveolus point. Because ventilation is equal from both alveoli, the mixed alveolar point will fall halfway between the two points at a mixed alveolar P_{O_2} of 125 mm Hg and a P_{CO_2} of 20 mm Hg.

Mixed arterial blood is a perfusion-weighted average of the blood coming from each alveolus. Because no perfusion comes from the dead space, the mixed arterial point must fall on a line connecting the normal alveolus point to the shunt point. In this case, the line is curved because the mixed point must be determined from the relative contents of blood from each alveolus, rather than partial pressures, even though the plot is on a partial pressure diagram. Because perfusion is equal from both alveoli, the mixed arterial point will fall approximately halfway between the two points (this would be exactly halfway if plotted on a content plot). The resulting arterial point has a P_{O_2} of 65 mm Hg and a P_{CO_2} of 42 mm Hg.

The new result reveals a very large difference between the arterial and mixed alveolar points. The alveolar–arterial P_{O_2} difference ($[A - a]P_{O_2}$) is 125 mm Hg − 65 mm Hg = 60 mm Hg, and the arterial–alveolar P_{CO_2} difference ($[a - A]P_{CO_2}$) is 42 mm Hg − 20 mm Hg = 22 mm Hg. These alveolar arterial differences are very large because a severely heterogeneous lung has been used for illustrative purposes. In the normal human, $(A - a)P_{O_2}$ varies from 10 mm Hg at 20 years of age to nearly 30 mm Hg at 70 years of age. The $(a - A)P_{CO_2}$ is quite small and is usually considered to be zero, even though the actual value is likely between 1 and 3 mm Hg.

A quantitatively more realistic example of a three-compartment representation of the normal lung is illustrated in Table 7.1. This lung has a low $\dot{V}_A/\dot{Q}$ alveolus, a normal alveolus, and a high $\dot{V}_A/\dot{Q}$ alveolus.

The mixed alveolar gas and mixed end-capillary blood P_{O_2} and P_{CO_2} can be determined from the conservation of mass principle. The mixed alveolar gas is weighted by the ventilation from each of the alveoli:

$$P_A = \frac{P_{A_1}\dot{V}_{A_1} + P_{A_2}\dot{V}_{A_2} + P_{A_3}\dot{V}_{A_3}}{\dot{V}_{A_1} + \dot{V}_{A_2} + \dot{V}_{A_3}} \tag{7.12}$$

Similarly, the mixed blood P_{O_2} and P_{CO_2} will be determined from a perfusion-weighted average of the O_2 and CO_2 contents from each of the three alveoli. The contents of each contributing blood stream must be used for calculation because we wish to keep track of all O_2 and CO_2 molecules.

$$Cc = \frac{Ca_1\dot{Q}_1 + Ca_2\dot{Q}_2 + Ca_3\dot{Q}_3}{\dot{Q}_1 + \dot{Q}_2 + \dot{Q}_3} \tag{7.13}$$

In the process of determining mixed alveolar gas, it is not necessary to use content because pressure and content are linearly related in the gas phase (but not in blood).

Table 7.1 shows the values used in determining the mixed arterial and alveolar P_{O_2} and P_{CO_2}. Arterial P_{O_2} (90 mmHg) is less than alveolar P_{O_2} (101.3 mmHg), whereas arterial P_{CO_2} (40.2 mm Hg) is greater than alveolar P_{CO_2} (39.6 mmHg). These relationships always hold, but the relative magnitude of the differences between alveolar gas and arterial blood increases as shunt or $\dot{V}_A/\dot{Q}$ heterogeneity increase. It is worth reiterating that the alveolar to arterial differences are affected by the relative matching of $\dot{V}_A/\dot{Q}$, but only slightly by the overall average $\dot{V}_A/\dot{Q}$.

Table 7.1. Three-Compartment Lung with Shunt and Dead Space

	COMPARTMENT			MIXED ALVEOLAR GAS	MIXED END-CAPILLARY BLOOD	SHUNT $\dot{V}_A/\dot{Q} = 0$	DEAD SPACE $\dot{V}_A/\dot{Q} = \infty$	MIXED EXPIRED GAS	MIXED ARTERIAL BLOOD
	1 $\dot{V}_A/\dot{Q}$	2 $\dot{V}_A/\dot{Q}$	3 $\dot{V}_A/\dot{Q}$						
$\dot{V}_A$ (l · min⁻¹)	0.4	3.0	0.6	4	—	—	2.0	6.0	—
$\dot{Q}$ (l · min⁻¹)	1.0	3.8	0.2	—	5.0	0.25	—	—	5.2
$\dot{V}_A/\dot{Q}$	0.4	0.8	3.0	—	—	—	—	—	—
P_{O_2} (mm Hg)	75.0	100.0	125.0	101.3	95.0	40.0	150.0	117.5	90.0
CO_2 (ml · dl⁻¹)	18.5	20.0	20.1	—	19.7	15.0	—	—	19.5
P_{CO_2} (mm Hg)	43.0	40.0	35.0	39.6	40.0	46.0	0.0	26.4	40.2
C_{CO_2} (ml · dl⁻¹)	50.0	49.0	45.0	—	49.0	51.0	—	—	49.1
P_{N_2} (mm Hg)	595.0	573.0	553.0	572.1	576.6	627.0	563.0	569.1	578.5
P_T (mm Hg)	713.0	713.0	713.0	713.0	711.6	713.0	713.0	713.0	708.7

On the O_2–CO_2 diagram (Fig. 7.9), mixing of gas from two units results in a mixed partial pressure of O_2 and CO_2, which falls on a straight line between the two alveolar points. If equal ventilations come from both alveoli, then the mixed point will be equidistant from each alveolar point. If more gas comes from one of the units, then the mixed point will move nearer to that alveolar point, but still be on the line connecting the two points. The same principle holds for blood mixing. Because of the nonlinear O_2 and CO_2 equilibrium curves, however, the line connecting the two alveolar units is curved. In the case of the lung illustrated in Figure 7.10, three alveolar units are mixed, so the mixed alveolar point (A) lies nearest to the unit with the highest ventilation. The mixed capillary blood point (c) lies nearer to the alveoli with the highest perfusion.

The arterial point (a) is further determined by the mixture of shunt blood ($\bar{v}$), which reduces P_{O_2} but barely changes P_{CO_2}. Alveolar gas (A) is mixed with dead space gas (I) to create mixed expired gas (E), which lies on a line connecting the

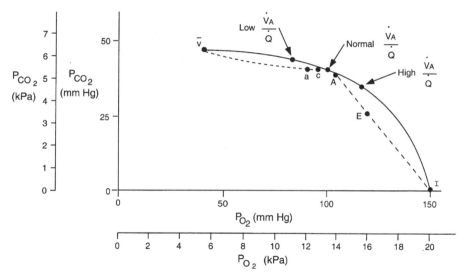

Figure 7.10. O_2–CO_2 diagram. A five-compartment lung with more realistic P_{O_2} and P_{CO_2} values. Three compartments with both ventilation and perfusion are shown as a low $\dot{V}_A/\dot{Q}$ unit, a normal $\dot{V}_A/\dot{Q}$ unit, and a high $\dot{V}_A/\dot{Q}$ unit. Mixed capillary blood is shown at c. Mixed alveolar gas is shown at A. C is mixed with shunted blood ($\bar{v}$) to yield mixed arterial blood (a). A is mixed with dead space gas (I) to yield mixed expired gas (E). (Adapted from Rahn H. A concept of mean alveolar air and the ventilation–blood flow relationships during pulmonary gas exchange. *Am J Physiol* 158:21–30, 1949; and Riley RL, Cournand A. 'Ideal' alveolar air and the analysis of ventilation–perfusion relationships in the lungs. *J Appl Physiol* 1:825–847, 1949.)

alveolar point and the inspired point. In a normal human, the shunt flow is less than 3% of the cardiac output, and dead space ventilation is about 25% of the total ventilation. Both of these values can change with disease, as can the relative heterogeneity of $\dot{V}_A/\dot{Q}$ distribution.

Closed Gas Volume Absorption

Closed gas volumes can be created in the body by a number of mechanisms: (1) trauma or chest wounds (such as from a bullet or knife) that introduce gas with a subsequent closure of the wound opening; (2) decompression sickness bubbles created by high concentrations of dissolved inert gas coming out of solution when exposed to a lower ambient pressure; (3) iatrogenic (caused by medical treatment) introduction of gas bubbles into the venous circulation during intravenous infusion; and (4) obstruction of an airway to a lung region that cannot ventilate via collateral ventilation channels. Any closed gas volume will eventually be absorbed by a complex diffusion process. The rate of this absorption, however, depends on a number of factors, including location of the gas volume, inert gas concentration in both the surrounding tissue and the gas pocket, relative perfusion to the surrounding area, and size and shape of the gas volume.

This situation can be understood by considering the analogous model of an occluded alveolus that is perfused by normal mixed venous blood but is suddenly unventilated due to blockage by a mucous plug. Immediately after the blockage, the alveolar gases are normal: $P_{A_{O_2}} = 100$ mm Hg, $P_{A_{CO_2}} = 40$ mm Hg, $P_{A_{N_2}} = 573$ mm Hg, and $P_{A_{H_2O}} = 47$ mm Hg. The total alveolar pressure is equal to barometric pressure (760 mm Hg), and the dry gas (minus water vapor) total pressure is 713 mm Hg. The total gas pressure* in mixed venous blood, however, is only 659 mm Hg: $P_{v_{O_2}} = 40$ mm Hg, $P_{v_{CO_2}} = 46$ mm Hg, and $P_{v_{N_2}} = 573$ mm Hg. The lack of equilibrium because of the mucous plug causes an exchange of gas. The flux of each gas is determined independently by Fick's law of diffusion (Eq. 7.1). Initially, there is a net outward flux of O_2 and an inward flux of CO_2. CO_2 diffuses in until the alveolar partial pressure reaches the $P_{v_{CO_2}}$ of 46 mm Hg and the flux stops. O_2 diffuses out, reducing the alveolar P_{O_2} below 100 mm Hg. Eventually, more O_2 diffuses out of the alveolus than the amount of CO_2 diffusing in, and the total volume of the alveolus becomes smaller. The negligible exchange of N_2 (because $P_{A_{N_2}} = P_{v_{N_2}} = 573$ mm Hg) along with the decrease in alveolar volume causes an increase in $P_{A_{N_2}}$ (the total pressure must equal barometric pressure) as the nitrogen fraction increases. The increase in $P_{A_{N_2}}$ (above mixed venous $P_{v_{N_2}}$)

---

*Water vapor pressure exists only in the gas phase, not in the liquid phase.

results in an outward flux of N_2 into blood. The concentrating effect increases PA_{CO_2}, reversing the movement of CO_2 to an outward flux. A steady process is achieved where partial pressures of all three gases are greater in the alveolus than in the blood, all three gases diffuse outward, and the alveolus gradually collapses, resulting in absorption atelectasis. This process can occur rapidly or take days, depending on the size of the occluded volume. If the patient is breathing 100% O_2 before the occlusion, there is no diluent N_2, and the absorption takes place much more rapidly.

Effect of $\dot{V}_A/\dot{Q}$ Heterogeneity on the Arterial–Alveolar Nitrogen Difference

Changes in inert gas concentration occur secondarily to exchange of the physiological gases, O_2 and CO_2. In low $\dot{V}_A/\dot{Q}$ alveoli, less CO_2 is added to the alveolus than the amount of O_2 that is taken up by the blood ($R = \dot{V}_{CO_2}/\dot{V}_{O_2} > 1$), decreasing alveolar volume. Because there is essentially no N_2 exchange due to its low blood solubility, the same number of N_2 molecules now occupying a smaller volume will contribute an increased N_2 partial pressure. For a high $\dot{V}A/\dot{Q}$ unit in which $R > 1$, more CO_2 will be added to the alveolus than the amount of O_2 taken up, causing a decrease in P_{N_2}. For a low $\dot{V}_A/\dot{Q}$ unit in which $R < 1$, P_{N_2} increases. The relative weighting of PA_{N_2} by ventilation and PA_{N_2} by perfusion makes PA_{N_2} greater than Pa_{N_2}. The magnitude of this $(a - A)P_{N_2}$ increases as the relative heterogeneity of $\dot{V}_A/\dot{Q}$ increases, and it has been used as a quantifier of $\dot{V}_A/\dot{Q}$ heterogeneity.

Functional Unit of the Lungs

The functional unit of an organ is the smallest structural element that can carry out the functional operations basic to the organ. In lungs, the functional unit is characterized as the smallest region within which there is gas exchange homogeneity—that is, diffusional equilibrium within the gas phase. The alveolus has been regarded as the unit of function by some investigators. The true functional unit is, however, very likely much larger than a single alveolus. The primary lobule, an alveolar duct and its alveoli and blood supply, form a unit because all alveoli of an alveolar duct are supplied by one pulmonary arteriole. It does seem more likely that the basic functional unit is larger than the alveolus—probably a cluster of alveoli associated with a last-order bronchiole in the conducting zone. The capillary networks of neighboring acini anastomose somewhat, but there is a distinct blood supply to each acinus. Even if there are separate capillaries within the functional unit with differing flow, the gas concentrations in the blood of each of those capillaries will be identical because of the diffusive mixing within the gas phase. The heterogeneity observed in gas exchange function can be attributed to differences in ventilation or perfusion of regions subtended by a terminal bronchiole. Studies of diffusion and convection show that, for all practical purposes, regions distal to the 16th to 17th generation airways (at the level of the respiratory bronchioles) are within diffusion equilibrium.

Arterial Hypoxemia

The gas exchange efficiency of the lung is the prime determinant of arterial P_{O_2}. Arterial hypoxemia has five causes:

1. Decreased $P_{I_{O_2}}$
2. Hypoventilation
3. Diffusion limitation
4. Shunt $\left.\phantom{\begin{array}{c}a\\b\\c\end{array}}\right\} \uparrow (A - a)P_{O_2}$
5. $\dot{V}_A/\dot{Q}$ heterogeneity

The first two factors, decreased $P_{I_{O_2}}$ and hypoventilation, affect Pa_{O_2} by reducing $P_{A_{O_2}}$. Neither shows an increase in $(A - a)P_{O_2}$. The last three factors, diffusion limitation, shunt, and $\dot{V}_A/\dot{Q}$ heterogeneity, increase $(A - a)P_{O_2}$ and result in arterial hypoxemia.

Clinically it is most important to determine the cause(s) of hypoxemia in a patient in order to provide optimal treatment. Decreased $P_{I_{O_2}}$ can be assessed by checking the inspired O_2 fraction (air or hypoxic gas mixture?) and noting the barometric pressure (altitude?). Hypoventilation can be assessed by measuring Pa_{CO_2}. Assuming $P_{A_{CO_2}} = Pa_{CO_2}$, an elevation in Pa_{CO_2} indicates hypoventilation and a subsequent reduction in $P_{A_{O_2}}$. A diffusion limitation can be assessed by measuring the lung diffusing capacity (see above). Diffusion limitation is rarely a problem except when there is a combination of decreased diffusing capacity (lung disease?), reduced pulmonary capillary transit time (exercise?), or reduced alveolar P_{O_2} (altitude?). Shunt can be assessed by measuring arterial P_{O_2} while the patient is breathing 100% oxygen. This eliminates the contributions of $\dot{V}_A/\dot{Q}$ heterogeneity and diffusion limitation to $(A - a)P_{O_2}$ and allows calculation of shunt (vide supra). The role of $\dot{V}_A/\dot{Q}$ heterogeneity is usually assessed by the process of elimination. If none of the other four factors is causing the observed hypoxemia, then $\dot{V}_A/\dot{Q}$ heterogeneity must be the culprit.

Further Reading

1. Farhi LE. Ventilation–perfusion relationships. In: Farhi LE, Tenney SM, editors. *Handbook of Physiology*, Section 3, *The Respiratory System*, vol IV, *Gas Exchange*. Bethesda, MD: American Physiological Society, 1987, pp 199–216.
2. Forster RE. Diffusion and convection in intrapulmonary gas mixing. In: Farhi LE, Tenney SM, editors. *Handbook of Physiology*, Section 3, *The Respiratory System*, vol IV, *Gas Exchange*. Bethesda, MD: American Physiological Society, 1987, pp 71–88.
3. Hlastala MP. Diffusing-capacity heterogeneity. In: Farhi LE, Tenney SM, editors. *Handbook of Physiology*, Section 3, *The Respiratory System*, vol IV, *Gas Exchange*. Bethesda, MD: American Physiological Society, 1987, pp 217–232.
4. Piiper J, Scheid P. Blood-gas equilibration in lungs. In: West JB, editor. *Pulmonary Gas Exchange*, vol I, *Gas Exchange*. New York: Academic Press, 1980, pp 131–171.
5. Wagner PD. Diffusion and chemical reaction in pulmonary gas exchange. *Physiol Rev* 57:257–312, 1977.
6. Wagner PD, West JB. Ventilation–perfusion relationships. In: West JB, editor. *Pulmonary Gas Exchange*, vol I, *Gas Exchange*. New York: Academic Press, 1980, pp 219–262.

Study Questions

7.1. Is it the partial pressure difference between alveolar gas and mixed venous blood or the β_m/β_b ratio that determines the rate of equilibration of a gas between capillary blood and alveolar gas?

7.2. Why is CO a suitable gas for measuring lung diffusing capacity?

7.3. List the three conditions that must be maintained to apply the 20 mm Hg $(A - a)P_{O_2} = 1\%$ shunt rule of thumb for estimating shunt.

7.4. Explain why gas emboli in the venous circulation will eventually be absorbed.

7.5. Explain why $\dot{V}_A/\dot{Q}$ heterogeneity has a much greater effect on $(A - a)P_{O_2}$ than on $(A - a)P$ of an inert gas.

7.6. Would increased $\dot{V}_A/\dot{Q}$ heterogeneity improve or worsen the washout of an inert gas by the lungs?

7.7. A patient arrives at a hospital emergency room short of breath. An arterial blood gas measurement taken while the patient was breathing air shows $P_{O_2} = 50$ mm Hg, $P_{CO_2} = 50$ mm Hg, and pH $= 7.32$. After placing the patient on 100% O_2 for breathing, an arterial blood gas shows $P_{O_2} = 363$ mm Hg, $P_{CO_2} = 51$ mm Hg, and pH $= 7.31$. A diffusing capacity test showed a DL_{CO} of 90% of the predicted value for the patient's age, gender, and height. Evaluate each of the five causes of hypoxemia to determine which are playing a role.

8

Central Mechanisms of Respiratory Control

Rhythmic contraction of the respiratory muscles produces the flow of gas into and out of the pulmonary system. Figure 8.1 shows the relationship between rhythmic, inspiratory phase–related bursts of electromyographic activity recorded in the diaphragm and the negative intrathoracic pressure generated by contraction of this primary muscle of inspiration. These events produce inspiratory tracheal gas flow and, ultimately, tidal volume expansion of the lungs. Rhythmic phrenic nerve activity emerging from the central nervous system (CNS) is the source of diaphragmatic electrical activity. Without the CNS, normal ventilation ceases, in marked contrast to the cardiovascular system, where the heart continues to contract and pump blood even when deprived of input from the CNS. Both the organization of CNS structures involved in rhythmic respiratory activity and ideas concerning the neural mechanisms responsible for respiratory rhythm generation are discussed in this chapter.

Voluntary versus Automatic Respiration

It is obvious that we can voluntarily alter our ventilation to meet the demands of speaking or breath-holding (e.g., when swimming underwater). Yet during various states of consciousness (e.g., during sleep) automatic ventilatory movements persist without the need for voluntary control. From these observations the concept of a dual control system has arisen, the system functioning separately for the most part and involving both voluntary and involuntary, or automatic, control of breathing. This dual system is most evident in humans and is clearly seen following high

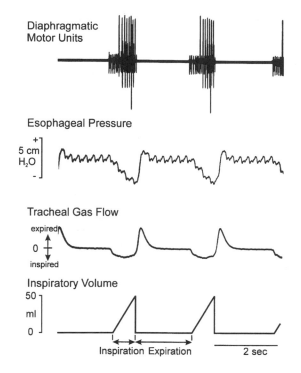

Diaphragmatic
Motor Units

Esophageal Pressure

+
5 cm
H₂O
-

Tracheal Gas Flow

expired
0
inspired

Inspiratory Volume
50
ml
0

Inspiration Expiration   2 sec

Figure 8.1. Rhythmic pattern of diaphragmatic motor unit discharge and its relationship to increases in negative intrathoracic pressure, inspired tracheal gas flow, and inspiratory lung volume. Esophageal pressure changes in the same direction by approximately the same amplitude during each breathing cycle as that of intrathoracic pressure. Small-amplitude, higher frequency waves in the esophageal pressure trace are due to cardiac movements. Data derived from anesthetized cat preparation. (From Berger AJ. Orderly recruitment of phrenic motoneurons. In: Binder MD, Mendell LM, editors. *The Segmental Motor System.* New York: Oxford University Press, 1990, pp 112–125, with permission.)

spinal cord lesions. For example, in the Ondine-Curse syndrome, which can develop after bilateral cutting of the ventrolateral cervical spinal cord for relief of pain, patients cannot make involuntary rhythmic breathing movements even when awake, but are able to breathe voluntarily when told to do so. During sleep such patients must be artificially ventilated. The spinal chordotomy in this case transected both ascending spinothalamic pain pathways and descending automatic respiratory tracts. Descending voluntary pathways to the respiratory muscles were, however, spared (see Fig. 8.6 later). The opposite situation involving partial transverse cervical myelitis has been observed. In this case, voluntary alterations in ventilatory movements cannot be accomplished, yet automatic rhythmic respiratory movements persist.

Humans do not normally perceive their breathing, and the perception of a shortness of breath or breathlessness is termed *dyspnea*. Dyspnea can occur in normal subjects, as during the ventilatory demands of heavy exercise. It can also be a symptom of heart and respiratory diseases. In these situations the perception is that the respiratory system is unable to meet the demands of O_2 delivery and CO_2 removal; thus the sensation of dyspnea may ensue. Recent evidence has indicated that dyspnea may result from the perceived mismatching of centrally generated respiratory movements from the demands placed on the respiratory system. Relief of the underlying disease state responsible for dyspnea is the overall goal of alleviating this symptom.

Organization of Brain Stem Respiratory Regions

Automatic control of respiration involves CNS structures in the pons, medulla, and spinal cord. Specific brain stem regions responsible for respiration have been localized in studies of experimental animals where the function of a brain stem region was inferred from alterations in respiration following destruction of the region. Figure 8.2 summarizes the results of these experiments, as well as the additional effects on the breathing pattern of transection of the vagus nerves. The vagus nerves (Xth cranial nerves) carry sensory neural activity from the airways and the lungs to the brain stem. When the brain stem is transected at level I, separating the pons, medulla, and spinal cord from more rostral CNS structures, the respiratory pattern is rhythmic and normal. When the vagus nerves are also cut, the inspiratory efforts are deeper (tidal volume [V_T] increases), are of longer duration (the duration of the inspiratory period is termed the *inspiratory time* [T_I], which increases in this condition), and are slower (*respiratory frequency* [f] decreases). These changes are consequences of release of the respiratory pattern generator from the effects of afferent fibers arising from sensory receptors in the airways and lungs (see Chapter 10). Increased tidal volume and decreased respiratory frequency also occur after bilateral vagotomy with an intact brain stem.

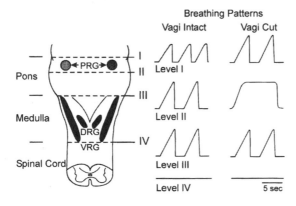

Figure 8.2. Breathing patterns observed following transection of the caudal brain stem at various levels before and after bilateral vagotomy. **Left,** Dorsal view of the caudal brain stem showing transections at levels I to IV and respiratory-related structures. **Right,** The breathing patterns observed with inspiration upward. DRG, Dorsal respiratory group; PRG, pontine respiratory group; VRG, ventral respiratory group.

These experimental results imply that afferent impulses, which arise from receptors in the airways and lungs and travel in the vagus nerves, act to limit the inspiratory tidal volume via a negative feedback mechanism. As the lungs expand during inspiration, these sensory receptors increase their activity. This neural activity is transmitted to the brain stem via the vagus nerves, where it provides an inhibitory influence on inspiration. The results showing continued rhythmic respiratory movements following vagotomy also support the concept that respiratory pattern generation can occur without sensory input from the periphery. Rhythmic ventilatory movements arise from a CNS pattern generator.

When the brain stem is transected at level II, in the middle of the pons, leaving the vagus nerves intact, tidal volume and inspiritory time are increased and respiratory frequency is reduced. This change in respiratory pattern is analogous to that which follows vagotomy. This provides evidence for the existence of a rostral pontine region, the pneumotaxic center, or *pontine respiratory group* (PRG) as it now is called, which functions to facilitate an earlier cut-off of inspiration. Thus, both the PRG and lung afferent inputs advance termination of the inspiratory phase of breathing. The PRG is composed of bilateral structures in the dorsolateral pons.

If brain stem transection at level II is combined with bilateral vagotomy, the breathing pattern is markedly altered. Inspiratory efforts are prolonged to a point where the observed inspiratory efforts have been called "inspiratory spasms" or "cramps"; this pattern of breathing is termed *apneusis* (a Greek word that means "holding of the breath"). Thus, in the absence of neural influences from the PRG and lungs, inspiratory time is markedly prolonged.

When the level of transection is moved caudally to separate the medulla from the pons (level III), a regular pattern of respiration again occurs. This pattern appears to be independent of ascending vagal influences. Finally, if a transection is made between the medulla and spinal cord (level IV), rhythmic respiratory efforts cease in the diaphragm and intercostals, the primary muscles of breathing. From these experiments in animals, it is inferred that the medulla contains the basic neural elements required for respiratory rhythmogenesis.

Respiratory Neural Structures Within the Medulla

Experimental findings have demonstrated that there are two dense, bilaterally organized longitudinal columns of neurons in the medulla, whose activity is directly related to various phases of the respiratory cycle. Figure 8.3 shows the locations of these neuronal aggregations, termed the *dorsal* and *ventral respiratory groups*. Within these groupings, there are various types of respiratory neurons.

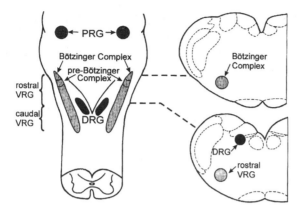

Figure 8.3. View of the pons and medulla showing the structures that have a high density of respiratory neurons. **Left,** Dorsal view of pons and medulla depicts the extent and anatomical designations of the structures. **Right,** Two transverse sections of the medulla showing locations of respiratory neuron-containing structures. Dashed lines indicate the rostral-caudal locations of the corresponding transverse sections. DRG, Dorsal respiratory group; PRG, pontine respiratory group; VRG, ventral respiratory group.

Ventral Respiratory Group

The ventral respiratory group (VRG) is located in the ventrolateral region of the medulla and is composed of a long column of respiratory neurons associated with several anatomically defined structures, including nucleus retroambigualis, nucleus ambiguus, and the pre-Bötzinger and Bötzinger complexes. The VRG is related to the phylogenetic development of respiratory structures. In fish, the branchial motor column, including motoneurons that rhythmically drive the muscles of the gills, is analogous to a part of this cellular column. There is reason to expect that an aggregation of respiratory neurons in mammals would be located at this ventrolateral medullary site. The VRG has both inspiratory (I) and expiratory (E) neurons. By definition, I neurons fire action potentials during the inspiratory phase of the respiratory cycle, whereas E neurons fire during the expiratory phase. Intracellular membrane potential recordings show that, during the same phase of the respiratory cycle, the membrane potentials of I and E neurons move in opposite directions. Thus the membrane potential of I neurons moves in a depolarizing direction during inspiration and in a hyperpolarizing direction during expiration, whereas E neurons are hyperpolarized during inspiration and depolarized during expiration.

I and E neurons are generally segregated within the VRG. At both the caudal and rostral ends of the VRG, E neurons are found in proportionately larger numbers; in the middle, I neurons predominate. Some VRG neurons have axonal projections within the medulla, and others project to more distant sites. For example, the motor innervation of the larynx arises from respiratory motoneurons whose cell bodies are located within the nucleus ambiguus portion of the VRG and whose axons are in the ipsilateral vagus nerves. Rhythmic respiratory-related movements of the larynx are readily observed. During inspiration the laryngeal opening dilates *(abduction)* and during expiration it becomes smaller *(adduction)*.

Many nucleus retroambigualis I and E neurons have axons that cross the midline of the medulla and turn caudally to descend into the cervical spinal cord. These provide rhythmic drive to phrenic, intercostal, and other spinal respiratory motoneurons. These inspiratory and expiratory systems are spatially separated, not only within the VRG but elsewhere: The axons from E neurons cross the midline caudally in the medulla, while the I neuron axons cross more rostrally; in the spinal cord the descending inspiratory and expiratory axonal tracts are spatially separated (see Fig. 8.6, later).

Recent evidence has indicated that the pre-Bötzinger complex is probably the site of respiratory rhythm generation. As discussed later, different mechanisms have been proposed by which pre-Bötzinger complex neurons generate this rhythm.

The E neurons concentrated at the rostral pole of the VRG, associated with the Bötzinger complex, provide widespread inhibition of several populations of I neurons. For example, they make direct synaptic inhibitory contacts with medullary I neurons and phrenic motoneurons. Thus, this pathway helps to ensure that I neurons will not fire during expiration.

Dorsal Respiratory Group

The dorsal respiratory group (DRG) is located in the dorsomedial medulla and is a subnucleus of the solitary tract, the longitudinally oriented fiber bundle within the medulla that contains afferent fibers of the glossopharyngeal and vagus nerves. This tract includes afferent fibers that arise from carotid and aortic body chemoreceptors, from slowly and rapidly adapting pulmonary stretch receptors, and from C-fiber endings in the lung. Not until the evolution of air-breathing creatures did the caudal portion of the solitary tract (as well as cellular aggregations associated with it) appear. This phylogenetic development is consistent with experimental observations that the caudal solitary tract region has a role in processing afferent inputs from the airways and lungs.

The DRG is part of the ventrolateral solitary tract nucleus and comprises a column of predominantly I neurons, although some E-neuronal activity can be found in this group of cells. I neurons are typified by two different patterns of activity observed in response to inputs from the lungs. Figure 8.4 shows schematically the neuronal classification scheme based on the different patterns. The *Iα neuronal type* has activity similar to the inspiratory motor output of the phrenic nerve. When the lungs are inflated synchronously with the motor inspiratory signal

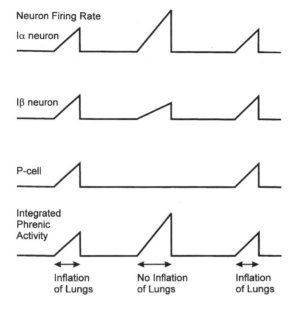

Figure 8.4. Neuronal classification scheme for the primary cell types within the dorsal respiratory group. Scheme involves different neuronal behaviors in response to withholding lung inflation (no-inflation cycle) during a period of augmented phrenic activity. Traces depicted show the neuronal spike discharge rates.

in the phrenic nerve, the Iα neuron shows a ramp-like increase in activity as inspiration progresses. When the lungs are not inflated, whether by occluding the trachea or simply not ventilating the paralyzed subject, an increase in peak phrenic activity occurs. This indicates release of inspiration from a feedback inhibition derived from the act of lung inflation itself (Hering-Breuer inflation reflex). Iα neuronal activity increases when lung inflation is withheld. Thus, both phrenic and Iα neuronal activities are inhibited by lung volume–related afferents.

The *Iβ neuronal type* has a response to lung inflation opposite that of the Iα neuron. Withholding inflation results in decreased Iβ activity (Fig. 8.4), indicating that lung inflation is excitatory to this cell type. Even without lung inflation, both the Iβ and Iα cells exhibit inspiratory activity, indicating that this activity arises from within the CNS.

The *P-cell type* does not exhibit a central inspiratory rhythm, but is activated by lung inflation–related inputs (Fig. 8.4). Because these cells do not have projections to the spinal cord, they are likely interneurons that have an important lung inflation–related sensory role. P cells closely mimic the behavior of the slow-adapting pulmonary stretch receptors (see Chapter 10). Afferent fibers from these receptors directly synapse onto P cells and thereby excite these neurons.

Many DRG neurons, including a large proportion of both Iα and Iβ neurons, have axons that cross the midline of the medulla and project into the contralateral spinal cord. It has been shown that these cells directly excite phrenic motoneurons and are in part responsible for the inspiratory-phase excitation of these important spinal motoneurons.

Respiratory Neural Structures Within the Pons

The PRG is the major concentration of pontine neurons with respiratory phase–related activity (Fig. 8.3). These neurons are concentrated in the nucleus parabrachialis medialis and Kölliker-Fusé nucleus of the dorsolateral pons. The PRG contains I-related and E-related neurons as well as an interesting class of neurons that have I–E phase-spanning activity that is not limited to either the I or the E phase of the cycle.

The function of the various respiratory neurons of the PRG is not precisely known. It may be that these neurons have a role in respiratory phase switching that influences the transitions between inspiration and expiration and vice versa. This idea is based on experimental results showing that electrical stimulation of the PRG can switch the respiratory phases, and destruction of this structure can markedly alter the breathing pattern (Fig. 8.2). The latter condition has also been observed in humans. Lesions of the dorsolateral pons, presumably involving the PRG, result in an apneustic breathing pattern in awake patients.

Spinal Cord Mechanisms of Respiration

Descending Pathways

The main muscles of respiration—the diaphragm and intercostal and abdominal muscles—are rhythmically activated by spinal α-motoneurons. Figure 8.5 illustrates the location of these α-motoneurons and the muscles they innervate. In humans, phrenic motoneurons form a longitudinally oriented column lying in the third to fifth cervical segments. Both internal (expiratory) and external (inspiratory) intercostal motoneurons form motor columns that extend the entire length of the thoracic spinal cord. The abdominal muscles of respiration, which have an expiratory function, have α-motoneurons occupying the lower thoracic and upper lumbar spinal cord segments.

The descending automatic respiratory drive to these α-motoneurons is carried in tracts that reside in the ventrolateral columns of the spinal cord (Fig. 8.6). Within the ventrolateral columns, the descending expiratory axons are situated medially,

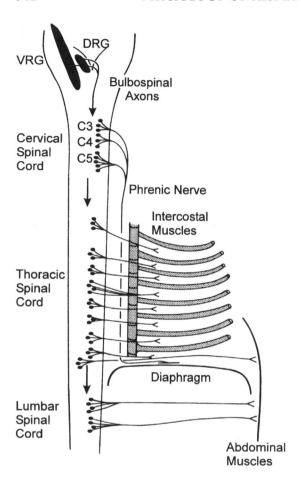

Figure 8.5. Illustration of the locations of phrenic, intercostal, and abdominal respiratory motoneurons in the spinal cord and their respective connections to respiratory muscles. DRG, Dorsal respiratory group; VRG, ventral respiratory group.

while the inspiratory axons occupy a lateral position. The tonic involuntary pathway is a second class of descending pathway originating in the medial reticular formation of the medulla. Although the function of this pathway is unknown, it may affect the average membrane potential of respiratory α-motoneurons. Modulation of the membrane potential by this pathway can influence the discharge pattern by placing the membrane potential of a motoneuron closer to or further away from its firing threshold. The descending spinal tracts for this pathway probably span the entire ventral column and a portion of the lateral column. Finally, descending tracts associated with voluntary control of respiratory muscles are located in the corticospinal tract in the dorsolateral portion of the spinal cord. Figure 8.6 summarizes the locations of these various descending pathways at the midcervical level.

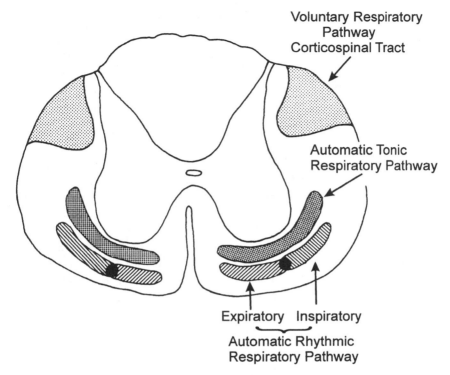

Figure 8.6. Descending fiber tracts for systems important in the control of spinal respiratory motoneurons. Depicted are the locations of the tracts at the midcervical level.

Integration at Spinal Cord Levels

Local spinal cord mechanisms are important to the activity of various respiratory motoneurons. In particular, the intercostal system has a higher proportion of γ-motoneurons than observed in the phrenic motor pool, consistent with the important dual role of the intercostals in both respiration and posture. Both α- and γ-intercostal motoneurons are rhythmically excited by inputs arising from supraspinal respiratory neurons. This rhythmic excitation of the γ-motoneurons enables them to activate and thereby produce contraction of intrafusal muscle fibers. This activity will cause the intercostal muscle spindle to detect with increased sensitivity the stretch of the parent extrafusal muscle fiber. The activation of γ-motoneurons constitutes an important servomechanism for the feedback regulation of muscle force and length. Therefore, the α–γ system may be important in stabilizing ventilation, even when different mechanical loads would lead to its alteration.

Intracellular recording of both phrenic and intercostal motoneurons has revealed two important aspects of their rhythmic activity. First, these cells are actively depolarized by excitatory inputs from the medulla during the phase of the respiratory cycle when they fire action potentials. Second, during the phase of the respiratory cycle when they are quiet (e.g., during expiration for inspiratory motoneurons), phrenic and intercostal motoneurons are actively inhibited. This active inhibition may prevent or lessen the firing rate of a respiratory motoneuron during its inactive phase.

Respiratory Rhythm Generation

A fundamental question is what is the neural basis for the CNS generation of respiratory rhythm in humans and other mammals? Although we do not yet know the full answer to this question, the necessary requirements for such a system are evident when one looks at the rhythmic activity of respiratory motoneurons. Figure 8.7 shows the neural discharges recorded from phrenic, external (inspiratory) intercostal, and internal (expiratory) intercostal motor axons.

First, overall respiratory activity consists of a sudden onset of discharge following a period of inactivity. Second, in the primary respiratory motor outflow there is a crescendo of ramp-like activity during the active phase. Third, immediately following the peak of activity, the discharge abruptly terminates, followed by a period of relative quiescence. Close examination of the phrenic nerve discharge shown in Figure 8.7 indicates that there is some residual activity that decreases following cut-off of the inspiratory burst. This low-amplitude, diminishing activity is called *postinspiratory activity*. For the most part, the overall pattern of rhythmic respiratory activity seen in respiratory spinal motoneurons is also evident in inspiratory and expiratory brain stem neurons. Therefore, any model of the respiratory rhythm generator must predict this type of behavior pattern.

Despite the fact that the specific cellular mechanisms responsible for respiratory rhythmogenesis are not completely known, several concepts that govern such a system have recently emerged. One such concept is depicted in Figure 8.8. The idea portrayed is that the respiratory rhythm seen in the motor output to respiratory muscles emerges from a system that sequentially transforms an underlying timing signal generated by the respiratory rhythm generator into neural activity of an appropriate pattern in the various respiratory motoneurons. Thus the rhythm generator acts much like a clock mechanism generating signals marking the respiratory phase (such as the start and end of each inspiration). These rhythmic timing signals are then interpreted by a pattern formation mechanism that produces a respiratory-phase envelope of neural activity (such as the ramp-like discharge that is observed in some inspiratory neurons). This fundamental pattern of activity is then used as

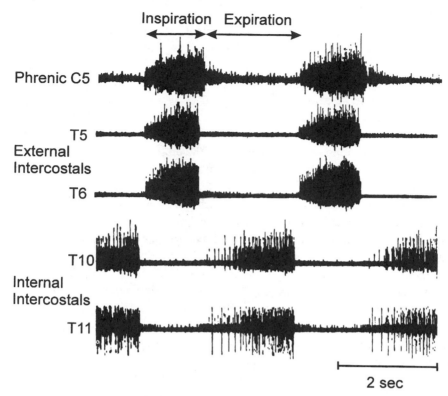

Figure 8.7. Spinal respiratory motor axon activities. Actual experimental record from an anesthetized paralyzed cat. **Top three traces,** Inspiratory motor activities (phrenic and external intercostals). **Bottom two traces,** Expiratory motor activities (internal intercostals). Intercostal activities recorded from the various thoracic segmental levels indicated.

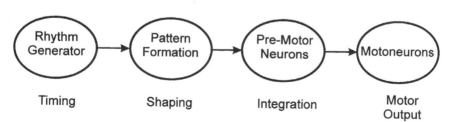

Figure 8.8. Schematic depicting the sequential steps in the transformation of a respiratory rhythm–generated timing signal into a respiratory-related motor output.

the major input to premotor neurons, which integrate various neural signals (such as respiratory-related reflex integration). Then, these premotor neurons provide direct synaptic inputs to the respiratory motoneurons themselves.

Concerning the rhythm generation mechanism itself, current thinking has narrowed the possible mechanism to two candidate systems. One system involves pacemakers, neurons that possess intrinsic properties associated with voltage and time-dependent ion channels, that are responsible for rhythmic behavior. Rhythmic activity in these neurons may be dependent on the presence of input systems, such as tonic excitatory inputs; these may be necessary to enable the neuron's membrane potential to be in a range where the voltage-dependent properties of the cell's ion channels result in rhythmic behavior. When such is the case, this pacemaker neuron is termed a *conditional pacemaker*. Recent *in vitro* studies have identified pre-Bötzinger complex neurons having voltage-dependent pacemaker properties, suggesting that they may be responsible for respiratory rhythm generation in this preparation.

Another system involves network interactions between neurons, that is, no single type of neuron on its own is responsible for respiratory rhythm generation. Interactions between neurons are required to generate rhythm. For example, reciprocal inhibition between I and E neurons may explain the absence of action potentials in one population of cells during its quiescent phase. This feature is bolstered by the observation that active inhibition during a neuron's inactive phase of the respiratory cycle is an underlying principle that appears to govern the behavior of many CNS respiratory neurons. I neurons are actively inhibited during expiration, and, conversely, E neurons are actively inhibited during inspiration.

It is unlikely that this is a general model for the organization of the system because *in vitro* studies have generally shown that following blockade of synaptic inhibition respiratory rhythm persists, and this occurs at all ages, yet *in vivo* data support the importance of inhibition in rhythm. Currently there is no resolution of this discrepancy, but one idea is that experimental conditions may cause different mechanisms of respiratory rhythm generation to be dominant; in the simplest case a pacemaker mechanism is dominant, while in more mature complex systems a type of hybrid model may be functioning. In this case the fundamental rhythm is generated by a pacemaker, but network interactions, including synaptic inhibition, are essential for the shaping and timing relationship that is seen in the respiratory motor output.

In summary, although we know a great deal about the respiratory neurons of the brain stem and the spinal cord, including their anatomy, inputs, outputs, and behavior, we still lack a complete understanding of the neural basis for respiratory rhythmogenesis. Nonetheless, recent studies with *in vitro* preparations are enabling us to begin to obtain new insights into respiratory rhythm generation.

Further Reading

1. Berger AJ, Bellingham MC. Mechanisms of respiratory motor output. In: Dempsey JA, Pack AI, editors. *Lung Biology in Health and Disease,* vol 79, *Regulation of Breathing,* 2nd ed. New York: Marcel Dekker, 1995, pp 71–149.
2. Bianchi AL, Denavit-Saubié M, Champagnat J. Central control of breathing in mammals: Neuronal circuitry, membrane properties, and neurotransmitters. *Physiol Rev* 75:1–45, 1995.
3. Feldman JL, Smith JC. Neural control of respiratory pattern in mammals: An overview. In: Dempsey JA, Pack AI, editors. *Lung Biology in Health and Disease,* vol 79, *Regulation of Breathing,* 2nd ed. New York: Marcel Dekker, 1995, pp 39–69.
4. Funk GD, Feldman JL. Generation of respiratory rhythm and pattern in mammals: Insights from developmental studies. *Curr Opin Neurobiol* 5:778–785, 1995.
5. Ramirez JM, Richter DW. The neuronal mechanisms of respiratory rhythm generation. *Curr Opin Neurobiol* 6:817–825, 1996.
6. Rekling JC, Feldman JL. PreBötzinger complex and pacemaker neurons: Hypothesized site and kernel for respiratory rhythm generation. *Annu Rev Physiol* 60:385–405, 1998.

Study Questions

8.1. Describe the change in the respiratory pattern when the vagus nerves are cut.

8.2. Describe the breathing pattern called *apneusis*.

8.3. Name the groups of respiratory neurons in the medulla.

8.4. How do P cells behave?

8.5. What anatomical structures make up the pontine respiratory group?

8.6. At what cervical levels are phrenic motoneurons located?

8.7. In which region of the midcervical spinal cord are the descending axons responsible for automatic respiration?

8.8. What are two cellular models that may be responsible for respiratory rhythm generation?

9

Chemical Control of Breathing

Hypoxia, hypercapnia, and acidosis are important stimulants to breathing. In this chapter sensory mechanisms that enable the body to detect each of these stimuli are described, and the overall ventilatory response to each stimulus is discussed.

Respiratory Response to Hypoxia

The respiratory control system responds with increased ventilation following the challenge of decreased PI_{O_2} and the consequent fall in Pa_{O_2}. The ventilatory response to hypoxia is due to the sensing of a reduction in Pa_{O_2} by sensory organs located on the arterial side of the circulation. Increased sensory nerve activity is transmitted to the brain stem where, following neural processing, this leads to an increase in discharge activity in nerves to the respiratory muscles. Ultimately, this increased discharge causes an increase in the output from respiratory muscles, thereby stimulating ventilation (Fig. 9.1). In this section we discuss this homeostatic feedback control system.

The Peripheral Arterial Chemosensors

The two groups of peripheral sensory organs responsible for detecting reductions in Pa_{O_2} are collectively called *peripheral arterial chemosensors* or *chemoreceptors*, the most important ones being the *carotid bodies*. Every individual has two carotid bodies located bilaterally in the neck at the bifurcation of the common carotid artery into its internal and external branches (Fig. 9.1). The blood supply to these small organs stems from branches of the carotid arteries. There also exists a second group of arterial chemosensors, the *aortic bodies*. The aortic bodies are located near the

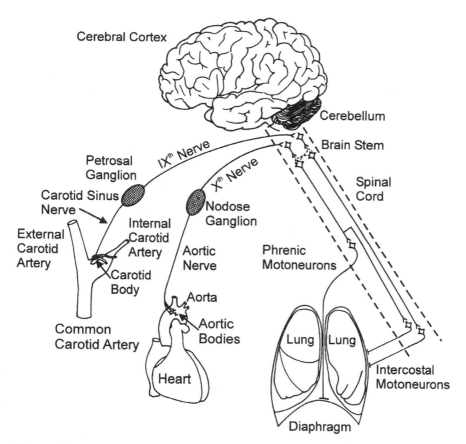

Figure 9.1. Schematic drawing illustrating the location of the neural pathways from the peripheral arterial chemosensors, carotid bodies and aortic bodies, and the central nervous system pathways that drive breathing.

arch of the aorta and receive their blood supply from small arteries arising from this large blood vessel (Fig. 9.1). In most respects, their function is similar to that of the carotid bodies. Because it has been found that the carotid bodies in humans are almost exclusively responsible for the ventilatory response to hypoxia, this chapter covers in detail only these sensory organs.

The carotid bodies have unique anatomical features. In humans, their extreme vascularity causes the carotid bodies to appear as small pinkish nodules that are approximately 5 mm long. Their arterial blood flow rate per gram of carotid body tissue is very high (approximately 20 ml $\cdot$ gm^{-1} $\cdot$ min^{-1}). Because this flow is high in relation to metabolism, there is little difference in the arterial and venous

O_2 partial pressures across these organs. Thus the small partial pressure difference allows the carotid bodies to be sensors of arterial blood gases (Pa_{O_2}, Pa_{CO_2}, and pHa) and to respond rapidly to changes in these variables.

The microscopic anatomy of the carotid bodies has led to several theories about how chemoreception occurs. Figure 9.2 illustrates some important structures located within a carotid body. The principal kinds of cells are *type I cells* (also called *glomus cells*) and *type II cells* (also called *sustentacular cells*) that surround or encapsulate the type I cells. Sensory nerve endings reside within the carotid body and have synaptic relationships with type I cells. These endings are the peripheral termination of sensory nerve fibers. The sensory nerve fibers emerging from the carotid body join sensory nerve fibers of the carotid baroreceptors to form the carotid sinus nerve. The cell bodies of this nerve are located in the petrosal sensory ganglion of the glossopharyngeal nerve (IXth cranial nerve). In addition, the carotid bodies contain autonomic nerves that regulate carotid body blood flow.

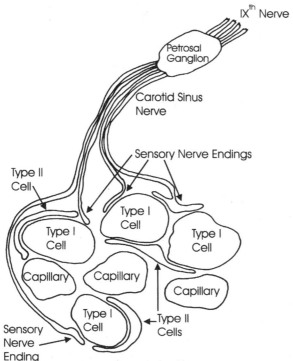

Figure 9.2. Schematic drawing of the cellular anatomy of the carotid body.

The present consensus is that the carotid body type I cells are responsible for sensing hypoxia. Type I cells have both pre- and postsynaptic associations with carotid sinus nerve afferent fibers. Recently, compelling evidence for a hypoxia-sensing mechanism in type I cells stems from biophysical experiments with voltage-clamp recordings that indicate that these cells possess an O_2-sensitive potassium channel. These experiments have shown that a reduction in P_{O_2} will reduce potassium currents in type I cells, thereby depolarizing them. In addition, type I cells exhibit increased action potential amplitude and increased firing frequency in response to hypoxia. This could cause an increased entry of calcium into the cells, which in turn increases the release of neurotransmitter-containing secretory vesicles. Type I cells have catecholamine-containing cytosolic vesicles that are secreted during hypoxia. Secretion of these vesicles is probably important in the signal transduction between type I cells and the nerve fibers.

Carotid chemosensory nerve activity is increased by a reduction in Pa_{O_2}; this response is nonlinear. Figure 9.3A illustrates the relationship between nerve activity and Pa_{O_2}. First, it shows that at normal levels of Pa_{O_2}, Pa_{CO_2} and pHa there is some carotid chemosensory nerve activity. Further more, even at hyperoxic levels of Pa_{O_2} ($Pa_{O_2} > 500$ mm Hg), there is low-level activity. Second, Figure 9.3A shows that as Pa_{O_2} is reduced from hyperoxic to normoxic to somewhat hypoxic levels, the nerve discharge rate rises only a small amount. Third, it is not until the level of Pa_{O_2} falls to approximately 50 to 60 mm Hg that activity markedly increases. As the Pa_{O_2} level falls further, the discharge activity continues to increase, reaching a maximum when Pa_{O_2} is approximately 20 to 25 mm Hg. Fourth (not illustrated), with further reduction in Pa_{O_2}, chemosensory discharge activity decreases, presumably due to detrimental effects of severe hypoxia on the sensory mechanism.

Based on experiments in which the carotid bodies were perfused with hemoglobin-free solutions and on other experiments in which hemoglobin in blood perfusing the carotid bodies was exposed to CO, it is apparent that the carotid bodies are sensing arterial Pa_{O_2} and not O_2 content. Therefore, if O_2 content is lowered while Pa_{O_2} is maintained, then carotid chemosensor activity will not increase. Thus anemia and CO poisoning, if not too severe, do not increase chemosensor discharge.

In addition to stimulation resulting from a reduction in Pa_{O_2}, the activity of the carotid chemosensory nerve fibers also is affected by Pa_{CO_2} and pHa (Fig. 9.3). Thus they contribute to the ventilatory response to hypercapnia and acidemia. If Pa_{CO_2} is increased at constant Pa_{O_2} and pHa (Fig. 9.3B), or if pHa is reduced at constant Pa_{O_2} and Pa_{CO_2} (Fig. 9.3C), then carotid chemosensory nerve activity increases. In summary, carotid chemosensors are sensitive to independent changes in Pa_{O_2}, Pa_{CO_2}, or pHa. It is important to remember that these chemosensors are considered primarily to be the sensors in the body's defense against hypoxia.

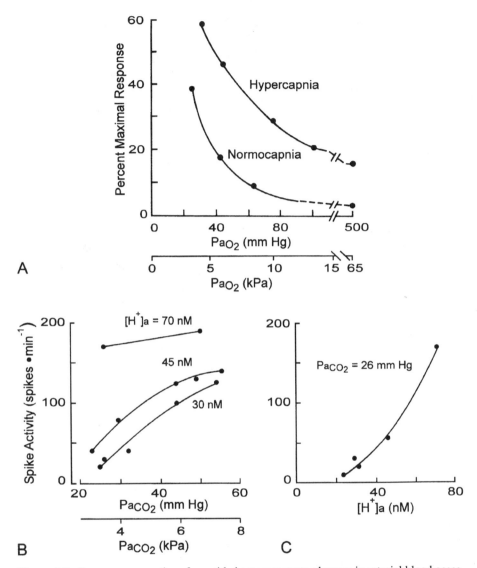

Figure 9.3. Response properties of carotid chemosensors to changes in arterial blood gases. **A,** Average response, as a percentage of maximal response, of carotid chemosensors to reductions in Pa_{O_2}, Data for normocapnia Pa_{CO_2} = 35 mm Hg and pHa = 7.33; data for hypercapnia Pa_{CO_2} = 57 mm Hg and pHa = 7.22. Data obtained from whole carotid sinus nerve recording in an anesthetized cat. (Based on data in Hornbein TF. The relationship between stimulus to chemoreceptors and their response. In: Torrance RW, editor. *Arterial Chemoreceptors.* Oxford: Blackwell Scientific Publications, 1968, pp. 65–78). **B,** Response of a single carotid chemosensor afferent fiber in an anesthetized cat to changes in Pa_{CO_2} at three different levels of $[H^+]_a$. Data obtained in a background of hyperoxia. $[H^+]_a$ maintained by altering $[HCO_3^-]_a$. **C,** Same as in **B** except response to changes in $[H^+]_a$ at a fixed level of Pa_{CO_2}. (**B** and **C** based on data reported by Biscoe TJ et al. The frequency of nerve impulses in single carotid body chemoreceptor afferent fibers recorded in vivo with intact circulation. *J Physiol [Lond]* 208: 121–131, 1970.)

Ventilatory Response to Hypoxia

As mentioned earlier, acute exposure to reduced $P_{I_{O_2}}$ stimulates ventilation due to sensory neural activity arising from the peripheral arterial chemosensors. Evidence for this includes the observation that in anesthetized cats a strong correlation exists between changes in carotid chemosensor activity, pulmonary ventilation, and Pa_{O_2} (Fig. 9.4). In humans, where the carotid bodies are almost exclusively responsible for the hypoxic ventilatory response, it has been found that when these bodies are surgically removed (a treatment used previously to lessen asthmatic bronchoconstriction), ventilation does not increase when $P_{I_{O_2}}$ is reduced. In this situation, as $P_{I_{O_2}}$ becomes low, ventilation actually decreases due to hypoxic depression of central nervous system function.

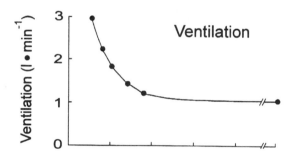

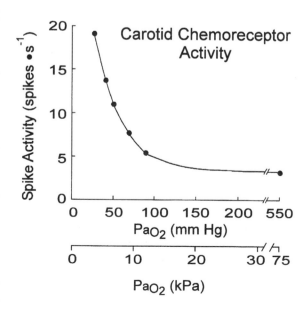

Figure 9.4. Response of ventilation and spike activity in a single carotid chemosensor fiber to changes in Pa_{O_2} recorded simultaneously in an anesthetized cat. The two responses correlate very strongly; both ventilation and chemosensor activity increase similarly with reductions in Pa_{O_2}. Data obtained under constant Pa_{CO_2} = 35 mm Hg. (Adapted from Lahiri S, Delaney RG. Relationship between carotid chemoreceptor activity and ventilation in the cat. *Respir Physiol* 24: 267–286, 1975.)

Figure 9.5A describes the normal ventilatory response to a decreasing Pa_{O_2} under isocapnic (fixed Pa_{CO_2}) conditions. Isocapnic conditions are maintained when a subject inhales small amounts of CO_2 as ventilation increases. Note that as Pa_{O_2} falls by 20 mm Hg from normoxic conditions (a Pa_{O_2} of approximately 100 mm Hg) to a slightly hypoxic level (a Pa_{O_2} of approximately 80 mm Hg), there is only a small increase in breathing. Only when Pa_{O_2} drops to approximately 60 mm Hg is a substantial increase in ventilation seen. Further reductions in Pa_{O_2} produce large nonlinear increases in breathing. At very low levels of Pa_{O_2} corresponding to severe hypoxemia, there is no further increase in ventilation, and this will eventually decrease because of the severe hypoxic depression of the central nervous system.

Several quantitative measures have been devised to assess a person's ventilatory sensitivity to hypoxia. This assessment is important for long-term residents of high altitude and for those patients with cyanotic congenital heart disease where the ventilatory response to hypoxia may be depressed. The isocapnic ventilatory response illustrated in Figure 9.5A can be quantified by the following expression:

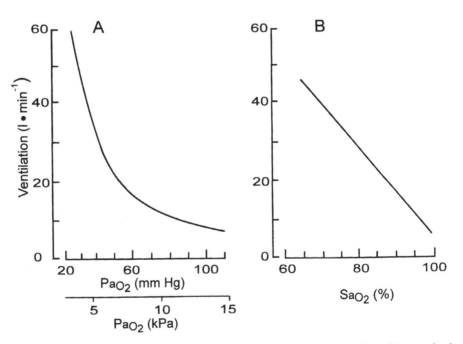

Figure 9.5. Average ventilatory response to hypoxia in a normal, awake subject under isocapnic conditions. **A,** Illustration of the hyperbolic relationship between ventilation and Pa_{O_2}. **B,** Plot showing linear relationship between ventilation and the percent arterial oxygen saturation (SaO_2). (Based on Berger AJ et al. Regulation of respiration. *N Engl J Med* 297: 92–97, 138–143, 194–201, 1977.)

$$\dot{V} = V_0 + \frac{A}{(P_{A_{O_2}} - 32)} \tag{9.1}$$

(Note that in Eq. 9.1, alveolar, and not arterial, P_{O_2} is measured because it is easier to measure, and the two values differ by the alveolar–arterial P_{O_2} difference.) Equation 9.1 is a nonlinear hyperbolic relationship between ventilation and $P_{A_{O_2}}$ and expresses the shape of the curve illustrated in Figure 9.5A. In equation 9.1, A is a measure of a subject's hypoxic ventilatory sensitivity: The greater the value of A, the greater the hypoxic sensitivity. There is wide interindividual variability in this value. A typical A value of about 185 l · mm Hg · min^{-1} has been observed in humans.

An alternative method of quantifying a person's ventilatory sensitivity to hypoxia is based on the experimental observation that, under isocapnic conditions, ventilation is a linear function of arterial O_2 desaturation (Fig. 9.5B). Thus, as O_2 saturation falls, ventilation rises proportionately. The ventilatory sensitivity to hypoxia can then be described as the magnitude of the slope of this relationship. The greater the slope, the greater the hypoxic ventilatory drive. Major benefits of this approach are that (*1*) rather than a nonlinear relationship (Fig. 9.5A), the variables of interest are linearly related (Fig. 9.5B), providing ease of calculation; and (*2*) arterial O_2 saturation can be measured noninvasively by using a pulse oximeter. On the other hand, hemoglobin desaturation in the absence of a fall in Pa_{O_2} (see Chapter 6) does not increase carotid chemosensory activity. Therefore, the relationship shown in Figure 9.5B is coincidental and does not reflect the underlying physiological mechanism responsible for stimulating breathing.

If isocapnic conditions are not maintained, hypoxia-induced increases in ventilation will cause a progressive fall in Pa_{CO_2} and a rise in pHa (*alkalemia*). This reduction in Pa_{CO_2}, with ensuing alkalemia, will attenuate the ventilatory response to hypoxia (Fig. 9.6; compare normocapnic and nonisocapnic responses). The mechanism for the attenuated ventilatory drive is a reduced sensory nerve activity from the carotid bodies (due to hypocapnia and alkalemia acting on carotid chemosensors) compared with its normocapnic condition. In addition, there is reduced excitation from another group of chemosensors located within the brain that are sensitive to changes in P_{CO_2}, central chemosensors (see later). Thus the overall effect on ventilation represents the central chemosensors "working against" the carotid chemosensors. The central chemosensors are functioning to depress breathing (brain alkalosis arising from hypocapnia), and hypoxia causes carotid chemosensors to stimulate breathing.

In contrast, if Pa_{CO_2} is not permitted to fall and isocapnic conditions are maintained, the resulting ventilatory response to hypoxia will be enhanced (Fig. 9.6, normocapnic). In this case, the central chemosensors are not exposed to reduced P_{CO_2} and therefore are not "working against" stimulation of breathing that arises from increased carotid body activity. Furthermore, carotid chemosensor activity will be greater because Pa_{CO_2} is higher and pHa lower than when Pa_{CO_2} is allowed to fall as ventilation increases.

Figure 9.6 also illustrates the ventilatory response to hypoxia when the level of Pa_{CO_2} is held at a constant elevated level (hypercapnic). Clearly, this ventilatory response is markedly enhanced and is not simply an arithmetic sum of the responses due to the hypoxia and the hypercapnia acting independently. It exhibits a multiplicative interaction, creating a ventilatory response larger than would be expected from a simple linear summation of the two stimuli.

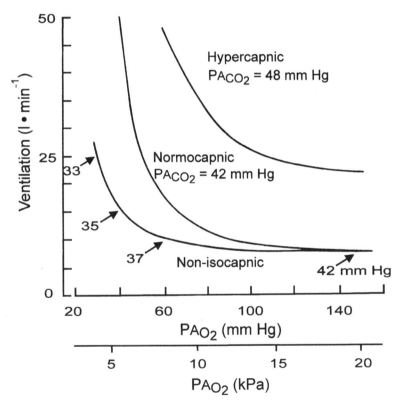

Figure 9.6. Ventilatory response to hypoxia in a normal, awake subject under different conditions of PA_{CO_2}. The **lower curve** illustrates the response when PA_{CO_2} is allowed to fall as ventilation increases with decreases in PA_{O_2} (values of PA_{CO_2} indicated at several points along the curve). The **middle curve** represents the isocapnic response (Pa_{CO_2} maintained at an approximately normocapnic condition of 42 mm Hg). The **upper curve** shows the response at elevated PA_{CO_2} (Pa_{CO_2} maintained at approximately 48 mm Hg). (Based on data reported by Loeschcke HH, Gertz KH. Enfluß des O_2-Druckes in der Einatmungsluft auf die Atemtätigkeit des menschen, geprüft unter Konstanthaltung des alveorlaren CO2-Druckes. *Pflugers Arch Ges Physiol* 267:460–477, 1958.)

Respiratory Responses to Carbon Dioxide and Hydrogen Ion

Increases in arterial P_{CO_2} and hydrogen ion concentration stimulate breathing. As with the ventilatory response to hypoxia, stimulation of breathing by CO_2 and hydrogen ion is a feedback control mechanism. The effects of changes in arterial P_{CO_2} and hydrogen ion concentration are considered together in this section. One reason we consider them together is because these two variables are linked via the Henderson-Hasselbalch relationship (see Chapter 13).

$$pH = pK + \log \frac{[HCO_3^-]}{[0.03 \times P_{CO_2}]} \qquad (9.2)$$

For example, equation 9.2 shows that when P_{CO_2} rises hydrogen ion concentration also rises (recall that $pH = -\log_{10}[H^+]$; therefore, when $[H^+]$ goes up, pH goes down).

Also discussed in this section are the alterations in breathing that occur both acutely (disturbances lasting seconds to minutes) and chronically (disturbances lasting hours or longer) in response to changes in P_{CO_2} and hydrogen ion concentration. The latter can occur in various disease states, such as CO_2 retention observed in respiratory failure and acidemia of diabetic ketoacidosis.

Central Chemosensors

If the peripheral arterial chemosensors are denervated (as when the sensory nerves from these structures are cut) and the inspired CO_2 level is raised to 3% to 5%, the subject will respond with an increase in breathing. This increase will be somewhat less than that seen when the peripheral chemosensors are intact. These observations led to the conclusion that the main site where increased CO_2 is sensed involves structures other than the peripheral arterial chemosensors, although these peripheral structures contribute somewhat to the overall ventilatory response to CO_2.

A search for sensory sites other than the peripheral chemosensors led Leusen in the early 1950s to perfuse the brain's ventriculocisternal system with an artificial cerebrospinal fluid (CSF) that contained elevated levels of hydrogen ion. This acidic perfusate produced an increase in ventilation. In the 1960s, Mitchell, Loeschcke, and colleagues showed that in experimental animals there is a region closely associated with the ventral surface of the medulla which, when acidified or when CO_2 is elevated, leads to an increase in breathing. More detailed studies following this initial discovery utilized various techniques such as lesioning, electrical stimulation, focal chemical application and cooling to reveal a more detailed mapping of this brain stem area. Based on this work, Figure 9.7 shows the location of chemosensitive areas close to the ventral surface of the medulla. There appear to

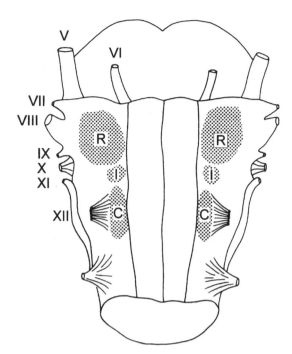

Figure 9.7. A ventral view of the medulla schematically illustrating the central chemosensitive areas (rostral, R; caudal, C). An additional intermediate zone (I) may have a function in central chemoreception, but its precise role is unclear. (From Berger AJ, Hornbein TF. In HD Patton, AF Fuchs, B Hille, AM Scher, R Steiner, Eds., *Textbook of Physiology,* 21st ed [revision of 20th ed, *Physiology and Biophysics*], vol 2. Philadelphia: WB Saunders, 1989, pp 1026–1045, with permission.)

be two bilaterally organized chemosensitive zones. One zone is located rostrally (area R) and corresponds to the region originally discovered by Mitchell, Loeschcke, and colleagues, and another zone lies more caudally (area C). An intermediate area (area I) lying between these two zones may also play a role in central chemoreception, but its precise function remains unclear. In addition to sites near the ventral surface, recent data have demonstrated that neurons more widely distributed in other regions of the medulla have chemosensory function.

The nature of the stimuli responsible for central chemosensitivity has also been investigated using *in vitro* preparations. For example, Figure 9.8 shows such an experimental preparation of the *in vitro* neonatal rat brain stem–spinal cord preparation that is capable of generating rhythmic respiratory-related neural activity in phrenic nerves (Fig. 9.8A). It is important to note that in this experimental preparation the lungs and muscles of breathing are no longer present, and respiration is inferred from the respiratory-like neural activity emerging from the central nervous system. When CO_2 is raised while hydrogen ion concentration is held constant in the perfusing fluid (by artificial elevation of $NaHCO_3$ as CO_2 is increased), the result is an increase in rhythmic respiratory-related neural activity (Fig. 9.8B). It is also possible with this preparation to hold the CO_2 constant while hydrogen ion con-

A

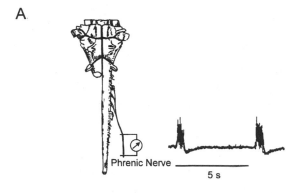

Phrenic Nerve ─────────
                5 s

B

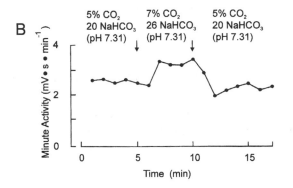

C

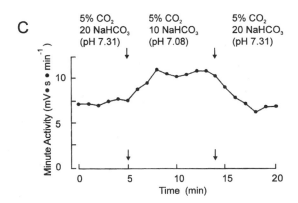

Figure 9.8. Effects of CO_2 and hydrogen ion on respiratory-related neural activity in the *in vitro* neonatal rat brain stem–spinal cord preparation. **A,** Schematic diagram of ventral view of lower brain stem and left half of spinal cord with recording of bursts of rhythmic neural activity from phrenic nerve. (Modified from Harada Y et al. Differential effects of carbon dioxide and pH on central chemoreceptors in the rat in vitro. *J Physiol [Lond]* 368: 679–693, 1985, with permission.) **B,** Effects of P_{CO_2} elevation at constant pH on respiratory minute activity. Changes indicated were made in the fluid bathing the preparation shown in **A. C,** Effects of pH reduction at constant P_{CO_2} on respiratory minute activity. In **B** and **C,** respiratory minute activity was determined from the peak amplitude of the burst of integrated phrenic nerve activity times the number of bursts per minute. Changes in respiratory minute activity are equivalent to changes in overall ventilation in intact *in vivo* preparations. (**B** and **C** from Harada Y et al. Central chemosensitivity to H^+ and CO_2 in the rat respiratory center in vitro. *Brain Res* 333: 336–339, 1985, with permission.)

centration is changed. As shown in Figure 9.8C, when the hydrogen ion concentration is increased without an increase in the CO_2 level (by artificial lowering of $NaHCO_3$), the result again is an increase in respiratory-related neural activity. Although these experiments show that independent increases in either CO_2 or hydrogen ion in the fluid bathing the brain stem are capable of increasing breathing, they do not provide information on the local CO_2 or hydrogen ion concentration at the central chemsensors themselves. Thus, in contrast to the peripheral arterial chemosensors, which have been identified as discrete anatomical structures and cell types, the specific cells that comprise the central chemosensors remain to be determined. This is necessary in order to definitively determine whether local hydrogen ion and CO_2 act as independent sensory stimuli. Local metabolism and transport mechanisms can modify CO_2 and hydrogen ion in the fluid surrounding the central chemosensors. Current research indicates that this fluid is the brain's extracellular fluid.

The Blood–Brain Barrier

Central chemosensors and central respiratory neurons are located within the brain and are therefore functionally and anatomically separated from any change in the constituents of blood by means of a structural arrangement termed the *blood–brain barrier*. Neurons in the brain are surrounded by extracellular fluid, the composition of which is governed by several factors, including brain cell metabolism, local

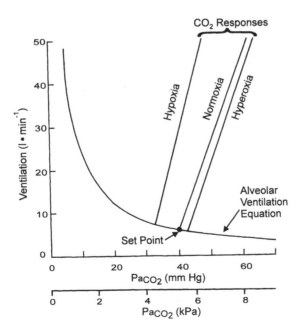

Figure 9.9. Linear ventilatory responses to changes in Pa_{CO_2} in three different background levels of arterial oxygenation. Also illustrated is the alveolar ventilation equation, which relates ventilation to Pa_{CO_2} (at constant metabolic production of CO_2), but in the absence of normal feedback control between ventilation and P_{CO_2}. The set point is the intersection of the alveolar ventilation equation and the normoxic ventilatory response, and it specifies the "normal" resting levels of ventilation and Pa_{CO_2}.

blood flow, and the CSF. Another characteristic of the brain's extracellular fluid and that of the CSF is that each is virtually protein free; therefore the bulk of the hydrogen ion buffering is due to bicarbonate.

An important feature of the blood–brain barrier is that it has low permeability to ions (such as hydrogen and bicarbonate ions) and high permeability to lipid-soluble molecules (such as CO_2). The selective permeability property of the blood–brain barrier has important consequences for the control of breathing. An example illustrates this point. Suppose that arterial hydrogen ion is quickly elevated by injection of an acid solution into the blood. If the degree of arterial hydrogen ion elevation is modest, the blood–brain barrier will prevent almost all of this increase from reaching the brain extracellular fluid, and the central chemosensors will not be stimulated. What actually happens is quite the reverse: The respiratory drive derived from the central chemosensors is diminished. The reason for this is that an increase in arterial hydrogen ion concentration can stimulate the carotid chemosensors, causing breathing to increase. The increase in breathing leads to a rapid fall in arterial P_{CO_2} because ventilation increases out of proportion to CO_2 production (recall Eq. 4.5 in Chapter 4 and see Fig. 9.9, the alveolar ventilation equation). Because the blood–brain barrier is highly permeable to CO_2, the reduction in arterial P_{CO_2} causes the normal flow of CO_2 out of the brain to increase, resulting in a decrease in the P_{CO_2} level within the brain. As a consequence of this acute lowering of the brain's P_{CO_2}, the hydrogen ion concentration within the brain's extracellular fluid also will fall (recall the Henderson-Hasselbalch relationship, Eq. 9.2). Thus, because of the blood–brain barrier, the elevation of arterial hydrogen ion in our example has produced a paradoxical effect: The carotid chemosensors are stimulated to increase breathing, but the drive that produces breathing, derived from the central chemosensors, is diminished (Table 9.1). The net effect is an increase in breathing that is somewhat attenuated.

Table 9.1. Chemosensory Contributions to Ventilatory Drive

	PERIPHERAL ARTERIAL CHEMOSENSORS	CENTRAL CHEMOSENSORS	OVERALL VENTILATION
Hypercapnia			
Acute	↑	↑↑↑	↑↑↑↑
Chronic	↑	↑↑	↑↑↑
Mild metabolic acidosis			
Acute	↑↑	↓	↑
Chronic	↑↑	O	↑↑

↑, ↓, and O indicate increase, decrease, or control levels of activity, respectively. Number of arrows and their length indicate relative contribution.

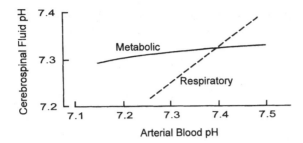

Figure 9.10. Cerebrospinal fluid pH versus arterial blood pH in chronic stable acid–base disorders. **Solid line**, metabolic acid–base disorders; **dashed line**, respiratory acid–base disorders. (From Fencl V. Acid-base balance in cerebral Fluids. In: Cherniack NS, Widdicombe JG, editors. *Handbook of Physiology. Acid base balance in cerebral fluids*, Section 3, *The Respiratory System*, vol II, part 1, *Control of Breathing*. Bethesda, MD: American Physiological Society, 1986, pp 115–140, with permission.)

If an elevation in arterial hydrogen ion is sustained, another interesting compensatory mechanism becomes evident. The hydrogen ion concentration of the brain's extracellular fluid will slowly increase and approach its normal value (Fig. 9.10). Therefore, the acid–base status of the brain is locally regulated, and the disturbances in the brain's acid–base balance are minimized over time. Several mechanisms for this regulation have been proposed: (*1*) active transport of hydrogen ion and bicarbonate ion across the blood–brain barrier; (*2*) passive distribution of hydrogen ion and bicarbonate ion, which relates to the electrical potential difference between CSF and blood (this difference in electrical potential varies with arterial hydrogen ion concentration); and (*3*) exchange of ionic components between brain cells and the fluid surrounding them. The latter mechanism involves cellular metabolism in the brain, which can vary with acid–base status to elicit close regulation of the brain's acid–base environment. Also, glial cells may be involved in cellular buffering similar to the way erythrocytes are involved in this function in blood. Whether any (or all) of these mechanisms is important in the long-term regulation of the brain's acid–base status is not completely understood.

Ventilatory Response to Carbon Dioxide

Acute Response

As previously mentioned, when arterial P_{CO_2} is elevated, breathing increases. A significant portion of this response is due to activation of the central chemosensors, with some contribution from the peripheral chemosensors to the additional respiratory drive. Both types of receptors are thus acting in concert to increase breathing (Table 9.1). As the level of arterial P_{CO_2} rises from its normal value of 40 mm Hg, ventilation increases linearly (as shown in Fig. 9.9). In normal individuals, the slope of this response line, when determined against a background of hyperoxia, varies from 2 to 4 $l \cdot min^{-1} \cdot mm\ Hg^{-1}$. Also plotted in Figure 9.9 is the so-called alveolar ventilation equation, which describes the relationship between ventilation and P_{CO_2} if ventilation is voluntarily varied. Its relevance here is that the intersection of the alveolar ventilation equation with the line describing the subject's ventilatory response to P_{CO_2} is termed the *set point* of the system. This set point represents the normal value of ventilation (about 6 $l \cdot min^{-1}$) and of Pa_{CO_2} (about 40 mm Hg). Figure 9.9 also shows ventilation to be very sensitive to small increases in arterial P_{CO_2}. In contrast, much larger decreases in Pa_{O_2} from normal levels (e.g., a decrease to a Pa_{O_2} of 80 mm Hg) produce little change in ventilation. Thus, it can be concluded that resting ventilation is governed more closely by Pa_{CO_2} than by Pa_{O_2}.

Pa_{CO_2} falls when a person voluntarily hyperventilates. Because respiratory drive is very sensitive to the level of Pa_{CO_2}, such a drop in Pa_{CO_2} can reduce respiratory drive to a point where the subject will become apneic (stop breathing). Apnea will then cause the Pa_{CO_2} level to rise gradually due to continuous metabolic production of CO_2. This will continue until a threshold level of Pa_{CO_2} is reached and breathing resumes. The ability to observe hypocapnic apnea and the apneic threshold depends on the individual's state of awareness. Hypocapnic apnea can be demonstrated during anesthesia when the subject's Pa_{CO_2} is reduced by means of mechanical ventilation.

The ventilatory response to CO_2 is also affected by the level of oxygenation of blood. As arterial blood becomes hypoxic, the slope of the CO_2–ventilatory response line increases (Fig. 9.9) because, under hypoxic conditions, the carotid chemosensors contribute greater ventilatory drive as the CO_2 level rises. Other conditions can also alter the CO_2 response line. For example, anesthetics, depressant drugs, and sleep usually will shift the response line to the right, causing Pa_{CO_2} to be increased at a given ventilation, and these also may reduce the slope of the CO_2 response line. Age also decreases the slope of the CO_2 response line. In contrast, the slope can be increased and the line shifted to the left by certain neurochemicals and drugs, including norepinephrine, progesterone, and salicylates.

The assessment of a person's ventilatory response to CO_2 is important in a number of diseases, including lung diseases such as chronic obstructive disease. These patients may have CO_2 retention and reduced CO_2 ventilatory responses. A subject's CO_2 ventilatory response can be measured by making stepped changes in inspired P_{CO_2} and waiting for a steady state to develop. The response is now commonly determined by using a nonsteady-state rebreathing method: The subjects breathe in and out of a bag containing a mixture of CO_2 (7% to 8%) in O_2 while their ventilation and end-tidal P_{CO_2} values are measured. End-tidal P_{CO_2} is measured with a continuous infrared CO_2 analyzer or a mass spectrometer. The last portion of gas exhaled is measured because end-tidal P_{CO_2} closely approximates the alveolar P_{CO_2}. As end-tidal P_{CO_2} increases, ventilation also increases. Ventilation is then plotted against end-tidal P_{CO_2}, and the slope of this line is the CO_2 ventilatory sensitivity, which is virtually identical to that obtained using the steady-state method.

Chronic Response

During chronic hypercapnia, hydrogen ion concentration is not as elevated, in either blood or extracellular fluid of the brain, as is observed in acute exposure to the same level of Pa_{CO_2}. The reasons for this involve regulatory mechanisms that help to maintain the acid–base status of blood and brain (see Chapters 11 and 13). These regulatory mechanisms cause the pH of the blood and of the brain to be less acidic and, as a consequence, the ventilatory drive arising from peripheral and central chemosensors will be somewhat lower than in an acute situation (Table 9.1). The independent stimulatory action of CO_2 on both carotid chemosensors (Fig. 9.3B) and central chemosensors (Fig. 9.8B) may provide much of the drive for the elevated ventilation observed in chronic hypercapnia. Also, as shown in Figure 9.10, during a state of stable respiratory acid–base disturbance, the pH of the brain will be directly related to that of the blood. Thus both peripheral and central chemosensors will be contributing to the ventilatory drive in chronic hypercapnia.

Another important consideration is the elevated levels of arterial P_{CO_2} that can be encountered during respiratory failure. A very high P_{CO_2} can result in a central nervous system narcosis, which has a depressant effect on ventilation. Consequently, under these conditions a large portion of the ventilatory drive may be derived from the peripheral chemosensors due to the concurrent presence of hypoxemia.

The opposite condition to chronic respiratory acidosis, that of chronic respiratory alkalosis, is seen in individuals living at high altitudes. This condition and its relationship to the control of breathing are discussed in Chapter 11.

Ventilatory Response to Hydrogen Ion

Acute Response

Metabolic acid–base disturbances involve the elevation of nonvolatile (i.e., not due to CO_2) acids or bases in the body. We have already discussed the acute ventilatory response to mild metabolic acidosis (see Table 9.1). The most important aspect of this response is that ventilatory stimuli are derived from stimulation of the arterial chemosensors, but, because of the ensuing hypocapnia and the presence of the blood–brain barrier, the central chemosensors are functioning to reduce the drive to breathe.

Chronic Response

Long-standing elevation in arterial hydrogen ion concentration of metabolic origin is observed clinically, as in diabetic ketoacidosis. Here, because of an increase in the cellular use of lactate over glucose, the arterial hydrogen ion concentration is increased. Figure 9.10 shows that, although the acid–base status of the arterial blood can vary widely, depending on the degree of chronic metabolic acid–base disturbance, the acid–base state of the brain does not vary much from normal due to local regulatory mechanisms within the brain. As a consequence of these regulatory mechanisms, in metabolic acidosis the subject's ventilation will initially increase over the course of several days while the acid–base status of the brain returns toward normal from its initial alkalemic state (Table 9.1). This progressive increase in ventilation will reduce arterial P_{CO_2} and will act as a partial compensation in the blood for the metabolic acidosis.

The above description of the role of peripheral and central chemosensors in acute and chronic metabolic acidosis applies to mild acidosis ($\Delta pHa < 0.1$). In severe metabolic acidosis, the peripheral chemosensors do not appear to be necessary for a ventilatory response, indicating that other factors are governing the response. A possible explanation is that the severe arterial acidosis effectively produces acidosis of the fluid environment surrounding the central chemosensors, and this will stimulate ventilation.

Further Reading

1. Bisgard GE, Neubauer JA. Peripheral and central effects of hypoxia. In: Dempsey JA, Pack AI, editors. *Lung Biology in Health and Disease,* vol 79, *Regulation of Breathing,* 2nd ed. New York: Marcel Dekker, 1995, pp 617–668.
2. Cherniack NS, Altose MD. Central chemoreceptors. In: Crystal RG, West JB, Barnes PJ, Weibel ER, editors. *The Lung: Scientific Foundations,* 2nd ed. Philadelphia: Lippincott-Raven, 1997, pp 1767–1776.
3. Gonzalez C, Almaraz L, Obeso S, Rigual R. Carotid body chemoreceptors from natural stimuli to sensory discharges. *Physiol Rev* 74: 829–898, 1994.
4. Lahiri S. Physiological responses: Peripheral chemoreceptors and chemoreflexes. In: Crystal RG, West JB, Barnes PJ, Weibel ER, editors. *The Lung: Scientific Foundations,* 2nd ed. Philadelphia: Lippincott-Raven, 1997, pp 1747–1756.
5. Nattie EE. CO_2, brainstem chemoreceptors and breathing. *Prog Neurobiol* 59: 299–331, 1999.

Study Questions

9.1. Which cell type in the carotid body is most likely responsible for sensing low Pa_{O_2}?

9.2. Indicate the direction of change in the arterial blood gases (Pa_{O_2}, Pa_{CO_2}, pHa) that will stimulate the carotid chemosensors.

9.3. Describe the relationship between ventilation and PA_{O_2}.

9.4. What happens to breathing if subjects had their peripheral chemosensors removed and inspired CO_2 was raised from the normal value of 0%?

9.5. Explain the role of the blood–brain barrier in the chemical control of breathing.

9.6. What more closely governs resting ventilation, Pa_{O_2} or Pa_{CO_2}?

9.7. Describe the response of the peripheral and central chemosensors to mild acute acidemia.

10

Airway and Lung Receptors, Reflexes, and Autonomic Regulation

The airways and lungs are richly endowed with sensory receptors. When activated, these receptors have marked effects on respiration and other body functions. Targets such as smooth muscle and glands, controlled by the autonomic nervous system, are reflexively regulated by these sensory receptors.

Each of us has experienced the striking consequences of activation of sensory receptors in the airways and lungs. You need only consider the inhalation of dust into the nasal passages, which results in a sneeze reflex. Furthermore, if dust is inhaled through the mouth, bypassing the filtering mechanism of the nasal passages, it can reach the larynx and trachea, thereby invoking a cough reflex. Both the sneeze and cough are defense reflexes designed to remove particles of dust from the upper airways and to protect the lungs from invasion by foreign material. Airway defense reflexes also include an important autonomic component that may involve alteration in airway smooth muscle tone and mucus secretion. Figure 10.1 depicts the locations of airway and lung receptors and indicates the many reflexes they evoke.

This chapter describes several important receptors present in the airways and lungs and the reflexes that they elicit. Autonomic regulation of the airways and the bronchial circulation are also discussed.

Receptors and Reflexes of the Upper Airways

The upper airways comprise the nose, the pharyngeal region, the larynx, and the extrathoracic region of the trachea. These structures contain many different types

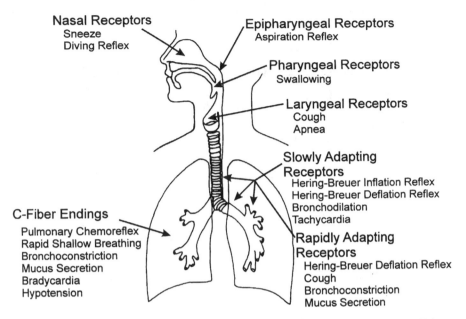

Figure 10.1. Location of major upper and lower airway and lung sensory receptors. Primary reflexes activated by these receptors are indicated.

of sensory receptors, which, when activated, lead to a number of distinct reflex responses. This section deals with some of the most important reflexes that are activated from receptors located in the upper airways.

Nose

Sensory afferent fibers from the nasal passages travel to the brain stem via the ophthalmic and maxillary divisions of the trigeminal nerve. The two primary reflexes initiated by stimulation of receptors in the nasal passages are the diving reflex and the sneeze.

The *diving reflex,* which can be elicited by water being instilled into the nose or applied to the face, encompasses a complex series of related responses involving the respiratory and cardiovascular systems. The former include a cessation of rhythmic respiration (apnea), closure of the larynx, and bronchoconstriction. The cardiovascular effects are also varied. They include a slowing of heart rate and vasoconstriction in some vascular beds, such as skin, muscle, and kidney, but not in others, such as the brain and coronary circulation. The main function of the diving reflex is to prevent water from entering the airways and to protect the vital organs (brain and heart) from the effects of apnea. This reflex is utilized routinely by diving mammals and ducks, but is also present in humans.

The *sneeze reflex* is invoked by stimulation of the lining of the nasal passages, such as by mechanical probing of this region, or by inhalation and deposition of foreign particles. Also, inhalation of gases that irritate the nasal passages can produce a sneeze reflex. The sneeze reflex involves a strong inspiration that is immediately followed by a vigorous exhalation. Most of the gas exhaled during a sneeze passes through the nasal passages. The function of this reflex is to clear the foreign material from these passages.

Epipharynx and Pharynx

The primary reflexes generated by stimulation of the epipharynx and pharynx are the aspiration, or sniff, reflex and the swallowing reflex, respectively. The walls of the epipharynx contain receptors that are sensitive to mechanical distortion. Thus, when the epipharyngeal wall is lightly tapped, an *aspiration reflex* is generated (Fig. 10.2A). This reflex is made up of a series of brief, strong inspiratory efforts. Functionally, this reflex causes material in the epipharynx to be dislodged and then to be moved into the pharynx from where it can be either coughed up or swallowed.

Activation of receptors within the pharynx can produce *reflex swallowing*. Swallowing involves the inhibition of inspiration, closure of the larynx, and the initiation of a complex series of coordinated muscular contractions that move material from the oral cavity into the esophagus. The inspiratory inhibition and laryngeal closure prevent material that is to be swallowed from entering the airways below the larynx.

Larynx

The larynx is highly endowed with many different types of receptors, and, correspondingly, it is the site of initiation of a large number of reflexes. An important class of laryngeal receptor is the *mechanoreceptors*, which are of both the slowly and rapidly adapting types. The mechanoreceptors have been divided into three functional classes: *pressure receptors*—those sensitive to either negative (collapse) or positive (distension) pressure within the upper airways; *drive receptors*—those sensitive to upper airway muscle contraction; and *cold receptors*—those sensitive to low temperatures. The pressure receptors are involved in an important reflex that is triggered by negative upper airway pressure. This reflex augments upper airway dilator (abductor) muscle activity, and this increased activity helps to maintain patency of the upper airways.

Other receptors are sensitive to irritant gases, such as ammonia, sulfur dioxide, and smoke. In addition, there is an important class of receptors that is sensitive to

A Epipharyngeal Aspiration Reflex

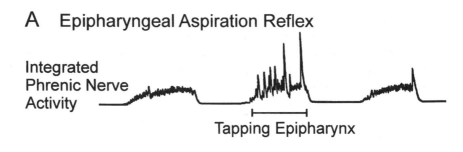

Tapping Epipharynx

B Laryngeal Apnea Reflex

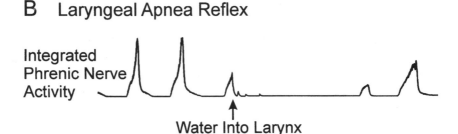

Water Into Larynx

Figure 10.2. Examples of upper airway reflexes. **A,** Epipharyngeal aspiration reflex produced by light tapping of the epipharynx. The result is brief strong inspiratory efforts, here indicated by large, short-duration increases in integrated phrenic nerve activity. **B,** Apneic response to injection of water into the larynx (at upward **arrow**). Apnea is shown as a prolonged, expiratory period (absence of integrated phrenic nerve activity) occurring immediately after water injectio. Experimental records in **A** and **B** obtained from different (anesthetized) cats.

water. Activation of receptors in the larynx can also produce a variety of reflexes, which include the cough and apnea. Figure 10.2B shows an apneic response to water application into the larynx. Note that immediately after introduction of the water there is a long-duration cessation of rhythmic respiration, indicated by the absence of rhythmic integrated phrenic nerve activity. This reflex is particularly evident in newborns and has been alleged to play a role in the sudden infant death syndrome (SIDS).

Receptors and Reflexes of the Lower Airways and Lungs

The receptors of the lower airways and lungs have been classified into two main types, each of which is further divided into two subtypes. The two main types of receptors are distinguished on the basis of whether the sensory afferent fibers are myelinated and therefore fast conducting or unmyelinated and therefore slow conducting. Regarding the anatomical projections of these afferent fibers, their primary pathway to the central nervous system for both myelinated and unmyelinated fibers from lower airway and lung receptors is via the vagus nerve. First, we discuss the two subtypes of receptors that transmit their sensory nerve traffic via myelinated vagal afferent fibers, the slowly and rapidly adapting receptors, and then we discuss the receptors that transmit via unmyelinated afferent nerve fibers, the pulmonary and bronchial C-fiber endings.

Slowly Adapting Receptors

The lower airways contain *slowly adapting receptors* (SARs) that are sensitive to mechanical distortion, that is, the stretching of an airway leads to increased activity of the receptors. In this way, these receptors are similar to the arterial baroreceptors, the latter being excited by stretching of the carotid sinus region by an increase in arterial pressure. Figure 10.3A, a recording of single sensory nerve fiber activity that arises from an SAR, shows that these receptors are excited by lung inflation, and the discharge slowly decreases (adapts) from its initial level; ultimately the discharge achieves a steady-state level in response to the increase in lung volume. The activity of these receptors progressively increases as lung volume increases (Fig. 10.4A). The primary stimulus to the SAR is an increase in tension of the airway wall. Many SARs are active even at the end of exhalation (at functional residual capacity [FRC]. The SAR appears to be located in close proximity to smooth muscle cells in both the extra- and intrathoracic lower airways. This location is supported by experiments that have shown SAR activity to change with bronchomotor tone.

The SARs are important components of several reflexes that cause changes in the pattern of breathing. One of the earliest described physiological reflexes, the Hering-Breuer inflation reflex, is elicited by activation of these receptors. Figure 10.5 (compare A and B) illustrates this reflex, wherein an increase in maintained lung volume during expiration markedly prolongs the expiratory phase of the respiratory cycle. This reflex constitutes negative feedback control of respiration because increases in lung volume serve to inhibit breathing. In addition to the effect of a steady-state increase in lung volume that inhibits breathing, lung inflation will progressively activate SARs even within a single inspiration, and this activation will curtail the inspiration. The latter effect helps to explain the respiratory pattern seen when the vagus nerves are cut (vagotomy), thereby removing the sensory input from SARs. Following vagotomy, inspirations (tidal volumes) are greater and breathing rate slows. Although changes in breathing pattern brought about by SAR activation can be easily demonstrated in some mammalian species, in humans they

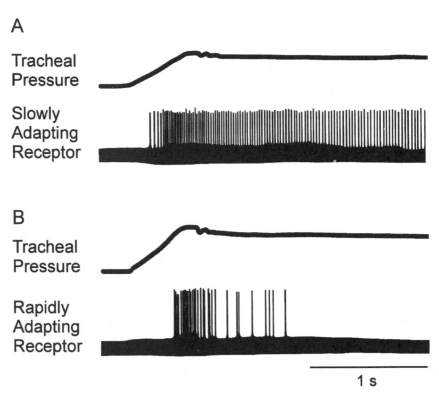

Figure 10.3. Responses to lung inflation (indicated by increased tracheal pressure in the upper traces) of a slowly adapting stretch receptor (**A**) and a rapidly adapting stretch receptor (**B**). In each case is shown a recording of a single afferent fiber dissected from the peripheral end of the vagus nerve (lower trace). Data from open-chested, anesthetized cat preparation. (Modified from Knowlton GC, Larrabee MG. A unitary analysis of pulmonary volume receptors. *Am J Physiol* 147:100–114, 1946, with permission.)

are not readily observed during resting tidal volume excursions. They do, however, become evident in all species, including humans, once inspiratory lung volume reaches higher levels (above resting tidal volume). In addition, activation of SARs has other reflex effects including bronchodilation and tachycardia.

Another interesting lung volume–related reflex is illustrated in Figure 10.5C: Lung deflation facilitates respiratory rate, shown here by the premature initiation of an inspiratory effort. This is called the *Hering-Breuer deflation reflex*, and it involves a reduction in activity in the SARs. The reason for this, as mentioned above, is that at FRC many SARs are active, and when lung volume is reduced from FRC the activity in these receptors is also reduced. This lessening of SAR

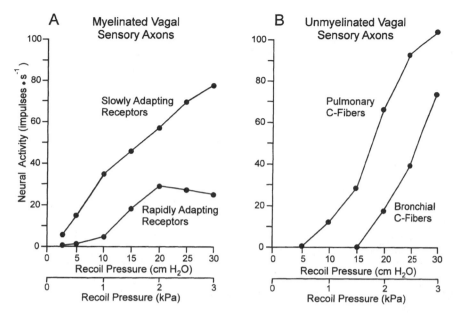

Figure 10.4. Comparison of the responses to a slow ramp of inflation for the four different types of lower airway and lung receptors. **A,** Response of slowly and rapidly adapting receptors. **B,** Response of pulmonary and bronchial C-fiber endings. The x-axis is trans-lung pressure obtained in open-chested, anesthetized dog preparation. Data points show mean values of firing rate. (Modified from Kaufman MP et al. Responses to inflation of vagal afferents with endings in the lungs of dogs. *Circ Res* 51:525–531, 1982, with permission.)

activity can increase breathing rate. A contribution to the Hering-Breuer deflation reflex by the rapidly adapting receptors (see below) is likely also, as these receptors are excited by lung deflation, and their excitation facilitates breathing.

Rapidly Adapting Receptors

The other subtype of receptor that transmits sensory nerve activity via myelinated vagus nerve afferent axons is the *rapidly adapting receptor* (RAR). There are fewer RARs than SARs. Also, their location is different, as they are associated with airway epithelium. Like the SAR, however, the RAR is considered to be primarily a mechanoreceptor, although it is also sensitive to various chemicals as well as to smoke and dust (which has led to the alternative name of *irritant receptor*).

The RARs are activated when the lungs are inflated quickly. If the lungs are held in an inflated condition, the RAR discharge shows both a profound and rapid

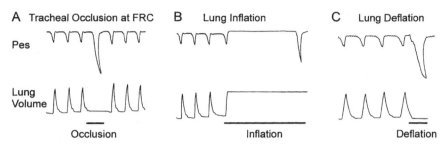

Figure 10.5. Effects of varying lung volume on respiratory pattern. Respiratory motor output monitored by esophageal pressure (Pes, where negative deflection is due to inspiratory muscle contraction) and lung volume measured by spirometer trace. **A,** Tracheal occlusion at functional residual capacity (FRC) has no effect on the time of onset of inspiration. Compare control expiratory durations before the occlusion with those during occlusion at FRC. **B,** Steady lung inflation by one tidal volume achieved by occluding the trachea at the peak of inspiration causes expiratory duration to be markedly enhanced during the steady lung inflation. This is the Hering-Breuer inflation reflex. **C,** Lung deflation by 100 ml, obtained by removing gas from the lungs at FRC and occluding the trachea. Expiratory duration is markedly shortened by lung deflation. This is the Hering-Breuer deflation reflex. Data obtained from anesthetized dog preparation.

adaptation; it ultimately ceases to discharge during long-duration steady inflations (Fig. 10.3B). This discharge also increases with both lung volume (Fig. 10.4A) and the rate of increase in lung volume, the latter reflecting the strong, dynamic sensitivity of the RAR. The lung volume at which firing begins is greater for RARs than for SARs (Fig. 10.4A). Another characteristic of these receptors is that they are also excited by large deflations of the lungs, and, as described above, they may be in part responsible for the Hering-Breuer deflation reflex (Fig. 10.5C). Finally, a reduction in lung compliance increases the discharge of RARs.

Both exogenous and endogenous chemical agents can cause excitation of RARs. In contrast to the rapid adaptation following mechanical stimulation, adaptation following chemical stimulation is slower. Among the agents that will stimulate RARs is histamine. Because histamine is endogenously produced, this has led to the idea that RARs may play a role in the reflex responses caused by certain lung pathologies, including asthma, where histamine is released in response to asthma-provoking challenges. Finally, it is still controversial whether the action of various agents on RARs is direct or is mediated indirectly by their effect on the receptor's local environment, which in turn would cause activation or sensitization of the RARs.

The reflex responses triggered by RARs seem to depend on the receptor location within the tracheobronchial tree. The RARs situated in the trachea and large bronchi are thought to be responsible for coughing, production of mucus, and bronchoconstriction. This triad of effects is functionally relevant. The cough is an airway defense mechanism the function of which is to remove offending material from the airways. It is a forced, rapid expiratory effort that creates high gas velocities that remove mucus from the airways. The offending particles are trapped in the layer of mucus that coats the airways. An increase in production of mucus aids the entrapment of foreign particles and thereby makes the cough more effective. Finally, bronchoconstriction, by decreasing the diameter of the airway lumen, increases gas velocity, further strengthening the efficacy of the cough.

C-Fiber Endings

Located within the lungs are receptors that send their sensory activity to the central nervous system via unmyelinated vagus nerve afferent axons, or *C-fibers*. These fibers have axonal conduction velocities of less than 2.5 m/s and constitute the vast majority of sensory fibers emerging from the lungs. The C-fiber endings can be divided into two types based on the vascular accessibility of chemical agents that excite them. Receptors excited at short latency after agents are injected into the pulmonary circulation (right heart injections) are termed *pulmonary C-fiber endings,* whereas those excited after a brief delay following bronchial circulation (left heart) injections are termed *bronchial C-fiber endings.*

Various exogenous and endogenous agents can stimulate C-fiber endings. It appears that the rate of infusion and dose of these agents influence the overall reflex response. Early observations indicated that activation of the C-fiber endings was responsible for the powerful, so-called pulmonary chemoreflex. This reflex involves both cardiovascular and respiratory effects: bradycardia, hypotension, and apnea, followed by rapid, shallow breathing (tachypnea). When high doses of chemical agents, such as capsaicin, the pungent ingredient of red pepper and paprika, and phenyl diguanide, a serotonin-3 ($5-HT_3$) receptor subtype agonist, are rapidly injected into the pulmonary circulation, they produce this reflex. Slower rates of injection and lower doses produce the same effects but without the preceding apnea. Some endogenous chemicals excite the C-fiber endings. These include histamine, bradykinin, serotonin, and prostaglandins. Because these naturally occurring agents can be released in certain pulmonary pathological states, such as in asthma, pulmonary congestion, or embolism, it entails more than academic interest that they excite C-fiber endings. The rapid shallow breathing associated with pulmonary pathologies may be due to pulmonary C-fiber ending activation.

In addition to their activation by exogenous and endogenous chemicals, C-fibers are also excited by lung inflation. At tidal volumes associated with normal quiet breathing, both pulmonary and bronchial C-fiber endings exhibit little activity. Although pulmonary C-fiber endings have lower lung-volume thresholds than bronchial C-fiber endings (Fig. 10.4B), lung hyperinflation excites both of these receptor subtypes.

Bronchial C-fiber endings may play an important role in reflex responses associated with airway defense mechanisms as well as those related to inflammatory reactions of the airway mucosa. Activation of these receptors induces an increase in airway smooth muscle contraction (bronchoconstriction) as well as an increase in airway vascular permeability. It is likely that release of neuropeptides from C-fiber sensory nerve endings themselves may be responsible for the local bronchomotor effects brought about by increased activity in these sensory fibers (see below). Evidence for this includes the observation that various neuropeptides are found in C-fiber sensory nerves of the vagus, and these neuropeptides are transported peripherally from the sensory cell bodies in the nodose sensory ganglion, where they are synthesized. The neuropeptide substance P has been implicated in this local reflex because it is present in sensory nerve fibers and it can cause bronchoconstriction.

Autonomic Regulation of the Airways

Autonomic control of the airways has cholinergic (parasympathetic), adrenergic (sympathetic), and peptidergic components. Table 10.1 summarizes these systems and the effects of each on airway smooth muscle tone. Other targets of autonomic inputs include mucous-secreting submucosal glands, vascular smooth muscle, airway epithelia fluid transport, and bronchial and pulmonary vascular permeability.

The airways are richly innervated by postganglionic cholinergic nerve fibers.

Table 10.1. Autonomic Components in Airway Regulation

SYSTEM	TRANSMITTER	RECEPTOR	EFFECT ON SMOOTH MUSCLE
Cholinergic	Acetylcholine	Muscarinic	Constrict
Adrenergic	Norepinephrine and epinephrine	β-Adrenergic α-Adrenergic*	Dilate Constrict
Peptidergic	Vasoactive intestinal peptide (VIP)	VIP	Dilate
	Substance P	Neurokinin	Constrict

* Note that direct α-adrenergic constriction of airway smooth muscle cells is observed only under special circumstances.

Adapted from: Barnes PJ. Neural control of airway function: new perspectives. *Mol Aspects Med* 11:351–423, 1990.

These fibers arise from parasympathetic ganglia located within the airways that are innervated by preganglionic parasympathetic fibers in the vagus nerves. The postganglionic fibers are important in the regulation of airway smooth muscle tone. To some degree, resting tone is due to activity in this system because cutting the vagus nerves or pharmacological blockade of the cholinergic system reduces resting airway tone. In addition, mucus secretion is enhanced by activation of cholinergic inputs to the airways.

In humans there is a sparser innervation of the airways by adrenergic (sympathetic) nerve fibers than by parasympathetic fibers. Postganglionic adrenergic fibers arise from sympathetic ganglia located in the paravertebral region. Overall, sympathetic activation leads to release of the neurotransmitter norepinephrine from these nerve fibers and to release of the circulating hormone epinephrine from the adrenal medulla. These have physiological effects, for example, on the state of smooth muscle contraction, through α- and β-adrenoceptor activation in target organs.

Postganglionic sympathetic fibers are closely associated with submucosal glands and blood vessels and also innervate the parasympathetic ganglia of the airways, but airway smooth muscle cells are poorly innervated by these sympathetic fibers. Even so, the sympathetic system can influence airway smooth muscle tone. For example, circulating epinephrine released from the adrenal medulla can activate β-adrenergic receptors on airway smooth muscle cells, and this can lead to bronchodilation. β-Adrenergic bronchodilation is the basis for the clinical use of β-agonists in the prevention and treatment of asthma. Selective $β_2$-agonists, such as albuterol and terbutaline, are used because they are less likely than β-agonists to have cardiac effects. There is evidence that α-adrenergic receptors are located in airway parasympathetic ganglia, and these can be activated by sympathetic nerve fibers. This activation inhibits cholinergic input to airway smooth muscle cells and thereby indirectly causes bronchodilation.

Neuropeptide-containing nerve fibers are present in the airways. These peptides are located in sensory nerve fibers of the C-fiber ending class and also in nerve fibers that appear to arise from parasympathetic ganglia in the airways. The latter component is called the *inhibitory nonadrenergic noncholinergic parasympathetic system* (i-NANC system), and activation of this system causes bronchodilation. One of the peptides associated with the i-NANC system and that has been isolated from the airways is *vasoactive intestinal peptide* (VIP). VIP has been shown to relax airway smooth muscle cells. Recent evidence has indicated that the transmitter nitric oxide (NO) functions as an important component of the i-NANC bronchodilatory response.

An *excitatory nonadrenergic noncholinergic* (e-NANC) response causes bronchoconstriction. This response involves release of tachykinins such as substance P contained in sensory nerve fibers (C-fibers) and activation of tachykinin receptors on airway smooth muscle cells. Release of substance P probably occurs via an axon reflex in C-fiber endings in the airways, and this may be one of the mechanisms by which C-fiber activation results in bronchoconstriction.

Autonomic Regulation of the Bronchial Circulation

The bronchial circulation is innervated by cholinergic, adrenergic, and peptidergic components. Bronchial blood vessels have a rich adrenergic nerve supply. The sympathetic innervation of these vessels produces vasoconstriction through activation of α-adrenergic receptors. Vasodilation results from activation of cholinergic and peptidergic mechanisms. In the latter instance both VIP and Substance P are potent bronchial vessel vasodilators.

Further Reading

1. Barnes PJ. General pharmacologic principles. In: Murray JF, Nadel JA, editors. *Textbook of Respiratory Medicine,* 2nd ed. Philadelphia: WB Saunders, 1994, pp 251–284.
2. Coleridge HM, Coleridge JCG. Reflexes evoked from tracheobronchial tree and lungs. In: Cherniack NS, Widdicombe JG, editors. *Handbook of Physiology.* Section 3, *The Respiratory System,* vol II, part 1, *Control of Breathing.* Bethesda, MD: American Physiological Society, 1986, pp 395–429.
3. Coleridge JCG, Coleridge HM. Functional role of pulmonary rapidly adapting receptors and lung C fibers. In: Lahiri S, Forster RE, II, Davies RO, Pack AI, editors. *Chemoreceptors and Reflexes in Breathing: Cellular and Molecular Aspects.* New York: Oxford University Press, 1989, pp 287–298.
4. Matran R. Neural control of lower airway vasculature. *Acta Physiol Scand* (Suppl 601) 142:1–54, 1991.
5. Sant'Ambrogio G, Tsubone H, Sant'Ambrogio FB. Sensory information from the upper airway: role in the control of breathing. *Respir Physiol* 102:1–16, 1995.
6. Widdicombe JG. Autonomic regulation: i-NANC/e-NANC. *Am J Respir Crit Care Med* 158:S171–S175, 1999.

Study Questions

10.1. What is the diving reflex?

10.2. Name the four major types of receptors in the lower airways and lungs.

10.3. Describe the Hering-Breuer inflation reflex, and name the receptor that is responsible for this reflex.

10.4. What triad of effects are rapidly adapting receptors in the trachea and large bronchi responsible for?

10.5. Describe the pulmonary chemoreflex, and name the receptor that is responsible for this reflex.

10.6. What is the effect of parasympathetic activity on airway smooth muscle tone?

10.7. What is the inhibitory nonadrenergic noncholinergic parasympathetic (i-NANC) system?

11

Respiratory Physiology with Altered Atmospheric Pressure

The respiratory system is well suited for excursions to, and even long-term habitation in, environments with altered atmospheric pressure. The adaptations that provide for this environmental flexibility are described in this chapter.

Response to Altitude

Ascent to altitudes significantly above sea level with its resulting hypoxemia initiates a number of mechanisms that enable humans to adapt to the adverse conditions encountered at such heights. This chapter describes the adaptive changes in response to the hypoxemia of altitude that occur in ventilation, in blood, and in pulmonary and tissue gas exchange, as well as the effects of altitude on exercise performance. These changes provide an integrative view of several concepts presented in earlier chapters.

Many of the adaptive mechanisms to sustained hypoxemia help to maintain delivery of O_2 to the body tissues. Figure 11.1 shows the relationships among barometric pressure, inspired P_{O_2}, alveolar P_{O_2}, and P_{CO_2} with respect to altitude. As altitude increases, PI_{O_2} decreases due to the fall in barometric pressure. Measurements in persons adapted to living at high altitudes indicate that alveolar P_{O_2} and P_{CO_2} both fall with increasing altitude, the latter being due to an increase in ventilation that is driven by hypoxemia.

There are limits to the human capacity for adaptive change to withstand the rigors of residing permanently at high altitude. The following two anecdotal examples give an indication of the altitude limit for permanent human habitation. In

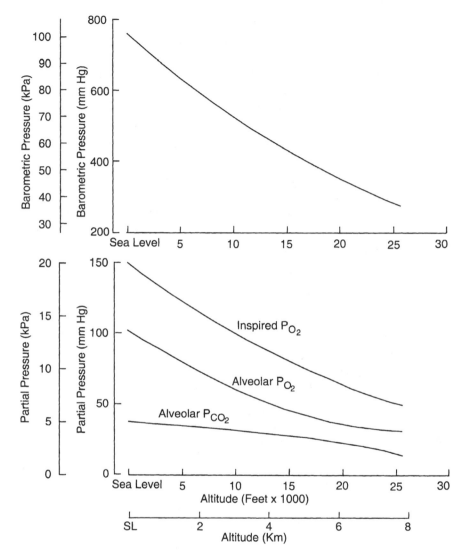

Figure 11.1. Relationships between barometric pressure, inspired P_{O_2}, alveolar P_{O_2}, and alveolar P_{CO_2} as a function of altitude. Alveolar gas compositions are derived from data from humans at altitudes, both acclimatized sojourners and permanent residents. Inspired P_{O_2} is for gas that is warmed and humidified to body conditions. (Data taken in part from those reported in Rahn H, Otis AB. Man's respiratory response during and after acclimatization to high altitude. *Am J Physiol* 157:445–462, 1949; and Pugh LGCE. Physiological and medical aspects of the Himalayan scientific and mountaineering expedition, 1960–1961. *BMJ* 2:621–627, 1962.)

the 1930s, D. B. Dill studied a group of sulfur miners living in a community located at an elevation of 5330 m (17,500 ft) in the Chilean Andes. The mine where they worked was 400 m above their village at an elevation of 5730 m (18,800 ft). These miners chose not to live near the mine head, presumably because of sleeping difficulties and problems associated with inadequate food intake. Each day they would climb from the village up to the mine. Another example of more recent origin also suggests that an altitude of 5730 m may be too high for permanent habitation. Pugh reported that during the 1960–1961 Himalayan Scientific and Mountaineering Expedition, a camp was set up at 5790 m (19,000 ft), which was inhabited for several months. It was found that all members of the Expedition lost weight while living at this elevation due to loss of appetite, suggesting that for nutritional reasons they could not remain at this altitude indefinitely. Thus the limit of permanent habitation for humans does not seem to be much higher than 5000 m even with the adaptations described below.

Ventilatory Adaptation

When an individual goes to a higher altitude, the most immediate effect is an increase in breathing. As shown in Figure 11.2, this acute effect is observed at elevations of 3000 m and above. This altitude corresponds to an inspired P_{O_2} of about 100 mm Hg and a $P_{A_{O_2}}$ of approximately 60 mm Hg (see Fig. 11.1). The immediate increase in ventilation arises from hypoxic stimulation of the carotid chemosensors. Over the course of the first few days, ventilation rises even more (Fig. 11.2). This time-dependent increase in ventilation in response to continuing hypoxemia is called *ventilatory acclimatization*.

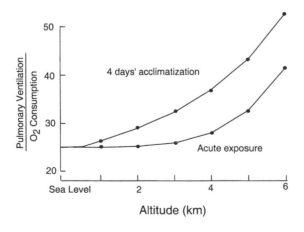

Figure 11.2. Relationship between ventilatory equivalent (overall ventilation/metabolic consumption of O_2) versus altitude both for acute response and after 4 days' exposure to hypoxia of altitude. (From Lenfant C, Sullivan K. Adaptation to high altitude. *N Engl J Med* 284: 1298–1309, 1971.)

Several important observations can be made with regard to ventilatory acclimatization. One is illustrated in Figure 11.2, where it can be seen that, although the acute increase in ventilation is not very evident at altitudes below 3000 m, after 4 days there is a discernible ventilatory increase at elevations as low as 1000 m. It is not clear why this difference exists.

A second important point can be drawn from Figure 11.3, where alveolar P_{CO_2} is plotted against alveolar P_{O_2} both for acute altitude exposure and after acclimatization. It is evident that at a given altitude the ventilatory increase with acclimatization produces an increase in alveolar P_{O_2} with a further reduction in alveolar P_{CO_2}. The increase in alveolar P_{O_2} with acclimatization is a beneficial adaptation; it occurs at the expense of a further reduction in alveolar P_{CO_2}. The reduction in P_{CO_2} will, of itself, produce alkalemia.

A third feature of increased ventilation observed with acclimatization is the finding that, if the hypoxia of altitude is acutely reversed by returning the acclimatized subject to normoxic conditions, ventilation will diminish abruptly, but it will remain elevated compared with its usual value at sea level. When the accli-

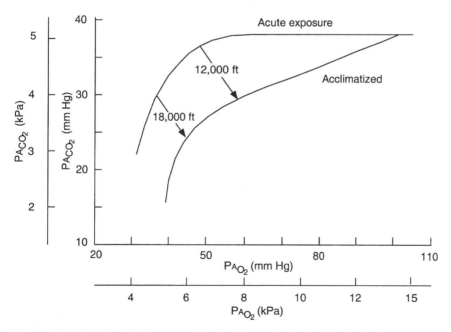

Figure 11.3. Relationship between alveolar P_{CO_2} and alveolar P_{O_2} for both acute exposure to altitude and following ventilatory acclimatization. Arrows joining the acute and acclimatized response curves are iso-altitude lines. (From Rahn H, Otis AB. Man's respiratory response during and after acclimatization to high altitude. *Am J Physiol* 157:445–462, 1949.)

matized subject returns to sea level, the process of deacclimatization begins, and ventilation gradually returns to its sea-level value over a course of hours to days.

The mechanism causing the ventilatory acclimatization process to occur is worth considering. One of the first hypotheses to explain the progressive increase in ventilation involved a return of pHa toward normal through renal compensation of the primary respiratory alkalosis. Bicarbonate ion excretion by the kidneys occurs in response to prolonged hypocapnia. This is an attractive explanation because of the known sensitivity of carotid chemosensors to $[H^+]_a$. Unfortunately, this mechanism cannot fully explain the progressive increase in ventilation that occurs. The reason for this is that renal compensation takes much longer than the increase in ventilation with acclimatization.

A second hypothesis concerns the ionic environment surrounding the central chemosensors. It was proposed that during the course of acclimatization there is a progressive acidification of the fluid bathing the central chemosensors compared with the alkalotic conditions present initially due to the increase in ventilation from hypoxemia. This acidification would cause the progressive increase in ventilation. The data, however, do not support this mechanism. Measurements of cerebrospinal fluid showed that following ventilatory acclimatization this fluid remained significantly more alkaline than normal. Without specific data obtained from the immediate environment of the central chemosensors (cerebrospinal fluid measurements may not provide this) it is difficult to rule out whether these structures contribute to ventilatory acclimatization.

A third and potentially more attractive hypothesis to explain ventilatory acclimatization involves a time-dependent increase in afferent neural activity from carotid (peripheral) chemosensors. Evidence for this includes the observations that in several species ventilatory acclimatization does not occur when the carotid chemosensors are removed. In the awake goat selective perfusion of the carotid bodies with hypoxic blood while the systemic circulation was maintained normoxic resulted in ventilatory acclimatization. The reverse situation of normoxic blood perfusing the carotid bodies in the presence of systemic hypoxia did not result in ventilatory acclimatization. Thus these studies provide evidence for an important role of the carotid chemosensors in ventilatory acclimatization. The specific mechanisms by which this happens, whether involving structural or neurochemical changes or changes in the O_2 transduction mechanism, remains to be established.

The above discussion concerns the ventilatory acclimatization that is observed in sojourners who go from sea level to altitude (days to weeks at altitude); long-term (years) residents at altitude exhibit a somewhat different ventilatory response. These individuals possess what is termed a *blunted hypoxic ventilatory response.* They exhibit a reduced ventilatory response to acute hypoxia. Also, compared with acclimatized sojourners to altitude, the ventilation of long-term residents at any given altitude will be somewhat less although significantly higher than in persons dwelling at or near sea level who experience acute exposure to the same degree of hypoxia. The mechanisms for this blunted hypoxic response as well as for the diminished ventilation at altitude are not known, but a number of adaptations do occur in humans residing at altitude that involve changes in blood and in pulmonary and tissue gas exchange. The changes may make it unnecessary for ventilation in long-term residents to be greatly elevated to ensure adequate O_2 delivery to the tissues.

Blood Adaptations

Hypoxemia increases the blood level of erythropoietin—a kidney-derived hormone that stimulates red cell production. The overall effect of this hormone is to increase both the hematocrit and the hemoglobin concentration in blood. This adaptive mechanism is very important because an elevated hemoglobin concentration enhances the O_2-carrying capacity of blood. A condition of polycythemia (increase in the number of red cells), however, is not without its own drawbacks because the viscosity of blood increases as hematocrit increases. After his visit to miners living at high altitude in the Chilean Andes, Dill vividly described this effect. He reported that arterial blood of one of the miners "was so viscous that the arterial pressure did not drive it into the syringe." The work of the heart is increased as blood viscosity increases. Thus a very high hematocrit level may actually be deleterious.

Another important blood adaptation involves shifts of the oxyhemoglobin equilibrium curve caused by elevated levels of 2,3-diphosphoglycerate (DPG) (which produces a rightward shift) and also hypocapnic alkalosis (which produces a leftward shift). Red cells produce increasing amounts of DPG in response to hypoxia. It appears that for subjects in a resting state at altitudes of up to 4250 m, the position of the *in vivo* oxyhemoglobin equilibrium curve for arterial blood is close to that observed at sea level. This is because there is a balance between the rightward shift arising from the increase in DPG and the leftward shift due to the hypocapnic alkalosis. In contrast, it has recently been observed that subjects in a resting state at extreme altitudes (above 6300 m) have a leftward shift of the *in vivo* oxyhemoglobin equilibrium curve due to an intense alkalemia arising from marked hyperventilation. The leftward shift with alkalosis is much greater than the smaller rightward shift due to increased DPG. The leftward shift of the oxyhemoglobin equilibrium curve enhances loading of O_2 in the lungs at very high altitude and thereby increases the O_2-carrying capacity of arterial blood.

Pulmonary Gas Exchange Adaptation

Several adaptive mechanisms help facilitate pulmonary gas exchange at high altitude. Two factors that determine the ability of the lungs to transport gases are the pulmonary diffusing capacity and the distribution of $\dot{V}_A/\dot{Q}$. High-altitude natives have an increased pulmonary diffusing capacity. This appears to result from an increase in total pulmonary surface area as well as an increase in pulmonary blood volume. The overall increase in pulmonary diffusing capacity enables the long-term resident to transport O_2 more effectively across the lungs. This mechanism is significant at altitude, where the rate of equilibration of pulmonary capillary P_{O_2} is reduced (see Chapter 7), but it would not play a role at sea level where in the resting state pulmonary capillary P_{O_2} equilibrates within one-third of the available transit time.

The efficiency of gas exchange is a function of the distribution of $\dot{V}_A/\dot{Q}$ in the various regions of the lung. The enhanced ventilation at altitude increases the overall $\dot{V}_A/\dot{Q}$ of the lungs and helps to raise the arterial P_{O_2} while lowering arterial P_{CO_2}. The matching of $\dot{V}_A$ and $\dot{Q}$, however, plays a greater role in determining arterial P_{O_2}.

Perfusion is also altered, but by a very different mechanism. Hypoxia at altitude causes pulmonary vasoconstriction. Figure 11.4 shows the marked elevation in mean pulmonary artery pressure as a function of altitude. This correlation is based on data obtained from persons born and permanently residing at various altitudes. Although this increase in pulmonary artery pressure has the negative effect of increasing the load on the right heart and therefore is maladaptive, it does promote redistribution of blood in the lungs, in particular causing greater perfusion of the lung apices and thereby causing a more uniform overall perfusion of the lungs. Despite observations of improvement in the overall perfusion distribution, recent gas exchange studies have shown that there is no enhancement in $\dot{V}_A/\dot{Q}$ matching with altitude.

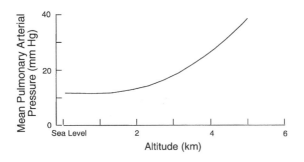

Figure 11.4. Correlation between mean pulmonary arterial pressure and altitude. Data obtained from subjects born and permanently living at various altitudes. (Based on correlation derived in Cruz-Jibaja et al. Correlation between pulmonary artery pressure and level of altitude. *Dis Chest* 46: 446–451, 1964.)

Tissue Gas Exchange Adaptation

The final step in the passage of O_2 from air to the blood to the tissues occurs in the tissue capillary beds. Analysis of skeletal muscle tissue from long-term residents at high altitude indicates that their capillary density is much greater. It is still uncertain whether this condition is due to generation of new capillaries, recruitment of previously closed capillaries, or both. The physiological implication of an increase in capillary density is a reduced diffusion distance between capillaries and cells where the O_2 is utilized. This would enhance O_2 transport to the cells (see Fig. 6.7).

Another adaptive mechanism involves an increase in the density of mitochondria with altitude. This is relevant for enhanced survival because the mitochondria generate adenosine triphosphate (ATP) from oxidation of sugars. Thus the higher density of mitochondria at altitude enables the scarcer O_2 molecules to be utilized more effectively to produce ATP. Thus energy production is less likely to be hindered.

Exercise Performance at High Altitude

Exercise during hypoxic stress at altitude reveals some of the limitations of these adaptive mechanisms. One of the most obvious limitations at altitude is the reduction of maximal O_2 consumption. Even though O_2 consumption at altitude is linearly related to work rate, as it is at sea level, it has been consistently observed that maximal O_2 consumption declines with increasing altitude (Fig. 11.5). Therefore, maximal work rate also declines with increasing altitude. Various factors are probably responsible for this diminution in maximal exercise performance. In contrast, one factor that would enhance exercise performance at high altitude is a

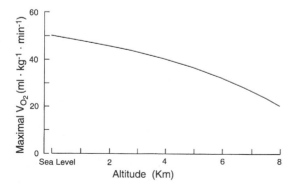

Figure 11.5. Relationship between maximum O_2 consumption and altitude for acclimatized sojourners to various altitudes. Note the reduction in maximum O_2 consumption with increasing altitude. (Based on relationship reported by Pugh LGCE et al. Muscular exercise at great altitudes. *J Appl Physiol* 19: 431–440, 1964.)

reduction in the density of inspired and expired gases. Reduced gas density would lower airway resistance and lessen the work of breathing at a given ventilation compared with that at sea level. This is a minor factor, however, that is only of some relevance at high altitudes. The overall effect of altitude is a reduction in exercise performance.

At high altitude, arterial O_2 saturation diminishes with increasing levels of exercise (Fig. 11.6). At very high altitudes the alveolar–arterial P_{O_2} difference may increase, and the difference widens further during exercise. This could be due to several factors, including increased shunt, $\dot{V}_A/\dot{Q}$ mismatch, and diffusion limitation. In exercise at high altitude, it appears that the most likely explanation for this widening of the alveolar–arterial difference is a diffusion limitation. First, there is a reduction in O_2 saturation leading to an increased effective O_2 solubility in blood (increased (β_b/β_m); see Chapter 7). Second, the elevated cardiac output of exercise— and therefore reduced residence time of blood in the pulmonary capillaries—fosters end-capillary disequilibrium (see Chapter 7). Third, during exercise, and particularly at altitude, there is a marked reduction in venous P_{O_2}; therefore, the amount of O_2 required to cross the pulmonary capillaries is very much increased (which causes a further increase in (β_b/β_m)).

Exercise performance at high altitude is diminished, but over time the adaptive changes in ventilation, blood, and pulmonary and tissue gas exchange help to improve this performance compared with that observed in the acute condition.

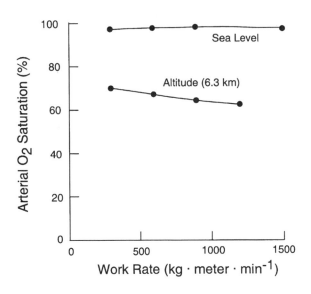

Figure 11.6. Relationship between arterial O_2 saturation and work rate at sea level and in acclimatized sojourners to high altitude (6.3 km). Note not only that the arterial O_2 saturation falls in subjects at altitude relative to sea level at all work rates but also that with increasing work the O_2 saturation falls at altitude but not at sea level. (Based on tabulated data reported in West JB et al. Maximal exercise at extreme altitudes on Mount Everest. *J Appl Physiol* 55: 688–698, 1983.)

Response to the Hyperbaric Environment

Excursion into a hyperbaric environment is becoming increasingly frequent for humans due to exploration and commercialization of relatively shallow regions of the sea near large land masses, the continental shelf. This exposure requires considerable ingenuity in adjusting to the many stresses related to the increased partial pressure of gases—both inert and respiratory gases—and the density-related changes in the mechanics of breathing.

Physics of Diving

Pressure is the force applied to a surface per unit of area. At sea level, the weight of atmospheric air results in an air pressure of 1 ATA (atmosphere absolute), which is equal to 29.92 in of mercury (in Hg), 760 mm Hg, 14.696 pounds per square inch (psi), or 750 kPa. When a person descends into water, pressure increases in proportion to the weight of the water and the air above. The density of water is such that pressure increases by 1 ATA for each 33 ft of sea water (fsw). Thus, at 66 fsw, pressure increases 2 atm above that at the surface, reaching 3 ATA. The relationship between depth and pressure is linear down to extreme depths because water is virtually incompressible (Table 11.1).

Boyle's law (see Chapter 1) demonstrates that pressure and volume of a gas are inversely related (pressure times volume is constant) at a given temperature:

$$P_1V_1 = P_2V_2 \tag{11.1}$$

At a constant temperature, a volume of a gas is inversely proportional to the pressure exerted on that gas. Consequently, when pressure doubles, the volume is re-

Table 11.1. Pressure versus Depth

| DEPTH (ft) | atm | ABSOLUTE PRESSURE | | | GAS PARTIAL PRESSURE | | | |
| | | | | | PI_{N_2} | | PI_{O_2} | |
		mm Hg	psi	kPa	mm Hg	kPa	mm Hg	kPa
0	1	760	14.7	75	564	75.2	149	14.7
33	2	1520	29.4	150	1165	150.4	308	30.4
66	3	2280	44.1	225	1766	174.3	467	46.1
297	10	7600	147.0	750	5974	589.5	1579	155.8
2250	69	52,440	1014.0	5175	41,443	4089.8	10,950	1080.6

duced by one-half. If a diver at 33 fsw (2 ATA) were to hold her breath and ascend to the surface, lung volume would double by the time she reaches 1 ATA, which could rupture the lungs if good diving practice (exhalation during ascent) is not followed.

Mechanical Limitations

The increased pressure of respired air causes increased density of air in the lungs, which has three primary effects. First, the inertance (inertial properties of gas molecules) of gas flowing through airways increases and may affect the distribution of ventilation. This effect of inertance is usually small, however, due to the small mass of gas volume, no matter how high the total pressure and density. Second, diffusion within the gas phase is inversely proportional to gas density, higher pressure reducing the relative mixing of inspired gas within the alveolar region. Third, increased airway resistance, due to the increased gas density, raises the work load required to achieve a given ventilation or can reduce ventilation at a constant work rate (Fig. 11.7). The increased work rate may lead to CO_2 retention at greater pressures as the diver reduces ventilation to avoid respiratory muscle fatigue. This reduced ventilation in response to increased work of breathing is similar to the response of the patient with severe chronic obstructive pulmonary disease (see Chapter 3).

Decompression Sickness

Normally, inert gas partial pressure in tissue is equal to that of the inspired air. When inspired inert gas partial pressure changes, due to a change in inert gas fraction or the ambient pressure, inert gases either diffuse into (*washin*) or out of (*washout*) the tissues. Each tissue is a well-mixed volume such that the washin or washout of inert gas is exponential in nature with a time constant depending on

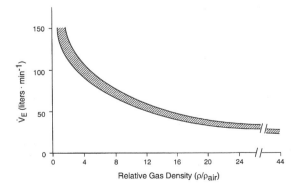

Figure 11.7. Maximum total ventilation versus increased depth plotted as relative gas density. (From Van Liew HD. Mechanical and physical factors in lung function during work in dense environments. *Undersea Biomed Res* 10:255–264, 1983, with permission.)

the volume of the tissue, the perfusion to that tissue, and the ratio of tissue solubility to blood solubility of the inert gas.

Decompression sickness (also known as the *bends* or *caisson workers disease*) can occur in divers after they ascend to the surface and are exposed to a reduced ambient pressure. This can also occur in pilots at high altitude and in astronauts during extravehicular activity. In all cases it is associated with a decrease in ambient pressure. Decompression sickness is caused by bubble formation in tissues and/or blood resulting from an initial exposure to elevated pressure and inert gas concentration with subsequent decompression and supersaturation of inert gases.

A diver descending to depth and breathing air at elevated pressure will inspire nitrogen at elevated partial pressure (P_{N_2}). Nitrogen equilibrates with various tissues of the body in an exponential manner, as shown in Figure 11.8. The curves in Figure 11.8 are actually a series of exponential curves connected together in time due to the sequentially changing partial pressure difference between the ambient and tissue pressures. The body has been described as having several tissues with differing half-times of equilibration. The faster absorbing (smaller half-time) tissues

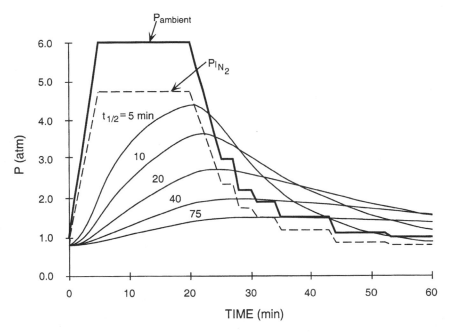

Figure 11.8. Schematic showing inert gas partial pressures in various tissues of a diver descending to a depth equivalent to 6 atm while breathing air and then ascending through a decompression profile. Inert gas partial pressure is shown in five tissues with half times ($t_{1/2}$) of 5, 10, 20, 40, and 75 minutes.

accumulates nitrogen more rapidly, and the slower absorbing (larger half-time) tissues will accumulate nitrogen slowly. After a fixed bottom time, the rapid tissues will be closer to equilibration with the nitrogen, while the slow tissues will have less nitrogen dissolved.

When the diver ascends to a lower pressure, inspired P_{N_2} is reduced. Rapid tissues with a greater P_{N_2} than inspired P_{N_2} begin to washout with a half-time of that particular tissue. The slow tissues with a P_{N_2} that is still lower than the inspired P_{N_2} will continue to washin nitrogen with their particular half-time, but with a smaller P_{N_2} difference. As the diver ascends further, following the decompression profile, the washout continues with identical half-times, but with reduced partial pressure driving force as the diver breathes progressively lower inert gas partial pressures.

In early diving research, Sir Charles Haldane found that divers could be compressed to 2 ATA for several hours and decompressed to 1 ATA with no apparent decompression sickness. He reasoned from these data that a 2:1 supersaturation ratio (the ratio between the pressure at which a diver breathes air to equilibrium and the pressure to which the diver is decompressed) was considered safe and caused no decompression sickness. Haldane concluded that divers could go deeper as long as decompression was controlled so that no tissues had more than a 2:1 supersaturation. He also recognized that the higher the degree of supersaturation, the more likely that bubbles would form and cause decompression sickness. Figure 11.8 shows that the relative degree of supersaturation in the various tissues changes during decompression. Early on, the rapid tissues are more supersaturated because they accumulated more nitrogen during time at depth. Later in the decompression, the rapid tissues washout and the slower tissues contain relatively more nitrogen because of their slower washout dynamics. The optimal decompression profile is one that minimizes the relative supersaturation of all tissues while minimizing the amount of time required for decompression. Identification of the best decompression profile has been the subject of great debate in the past two decades.

Gas Bubble Growth and Resolution

When a diver decompresses without allowing adequate time for inert gases to washout of all tissues, some regions may become supersaturated with inert gas and may trigger the development of gas bubbles, which cause tissue distention and the resulting pain of decompression sickness. The dynamics of growth or decay of an *in vivo* gas bubble play a major role in the development of decompression sickness. These dynamics are determined by the rate of gas diffusion into or out of the bubble. Because gas diffusion is determined by the partial pressure difference of that gas, the relative partial pressure of a gas within the gas phase of the bubble compared with the dissolved gas partial pressure in the surrounding tissue will determine the direction of gas diffusion. If gas is diffusing into the bubble, it will grow. If gas is diffusing out of the bubble, it will resolve (diminish and disappear). The overall growth or decay of the bubble depends on the sum of the flux of all gases in the bubble, each of which diffuses independently.

Under ordinary conditions, the sum of the partial pressures of all gases is greater within the bubble than it is in the surrounding tissue (see Chapter 7, closed gas volumes). Therefore, any gas phase within the body will normally resolve. In the gas phase in the alveoli, the sum of partial pressures of the gases is equal to atmospheric pressure (760 mm Hg under standard conditions at sea level):

$$P_{atm} = P_{N_2} + P_{O_2} + P_{CO_2} + P_{H_2O} \qquad (11.2)$$

$\dot{V}_A/\dot{Q}$ heterogeneity and normal shunt in the lungs causes arterial blood to have slightly lower total gas partial pressure than alveolar gas in the lung (see Table 7.1). As blood passes through tissue, delivering O_2 and taking up CO_2, further changes occur. Normally the respiratory quotient ($\dot{V}_{CO_2}/\dot{V}_{O_2}$) is about 0.8, meaning that 10 volumes of O_2 are delivered for every 8 volumes of CO_2 taken up. In addition, the effective solubility of CO_2 is greater than that of O_2. The net effect is a total partial pressure of O_2 and CO_2 in venous blood (40 + 46 = 86 mm Hg) that is less than the total in arterial blood (90 + 40 = 130 mm Hg). Tissue partial pressures of gas are closer to venous blood than to arterial blood partial pressures. The fact that a gas phase total partial pressure is greater than a tissue total partial pressure implies a net driving force for gas diffusion out of the bubble and a tendency for gas bubbles to resolve in any tissue.

If an air bubble (79% N_2, 21% O_2; P_{O_2} = 160 mm Hg, P_{N_2} = 600 mm Hg) were suddenly injected into the venous circulation, gas exchange with venous blood (P_{O_2} = 40 mm Hg, P_{CO_2} = 46 mm Hg, P_{N_2} eq 570 mm Hg) would occur. Gradients for O_2 and N_2 would diffuse outward (bubble to blood), and CO_2 and H_2O would diffuse inward (blood to bubble). The bubble would then be humidified via vaporization of water from the bubble surface, diluting the bubble "dry" gases and yielding P_{O_2} = 150 mm Hg, P_{N_2} = 563 mm Hg and P_{H_2O} = 47 mm Hg. At this point, there would be outward diffusion gradients for O_2 and inward gradients for CO_2 and N_2. Soon after, CO_2 would reach equilibrium and stop exchanging. O_2 efflux could continue at a rapid pace because of the relatively high solubility of O_2 in blood (this high solubility is even more characteristic of CO_2). The rapid efflux of O_2 and relative stoppage of CO_2 flux concentrates N_2 within the bubble because the sum of the partial pressures of all gases must equal total pressure (assumed to be 760 mm Hg in this example). This reestablishes an elevated bubble P_{N_2} and an outward diffusion of N_2. Eventually a steady state is reached where outward diffusive partial pressure driving gradients would be related by the inverse of the blood solubility times diffusivity of each gas (Fick's first law of diffusion), and the sum of partial pressures of each gas in the bubble would equal total pressure. Typical bubble gas pressures during this steady resolution process are P_{O_2} = 43 mm Hg, P_{CO_2} = 47 mm Hg; P_{N_2} = 623 mm Hg; P_{H_2O} = 47 mm Hg; compared with blood gases of P_{O_2} = 40 mm Hg; P_{CO_2} = 46 mm Hg; P_{N_2} = 563 mm Hg). Note that the partial pressure of each gas is higher in the bubble than in the blood during this resolution process. The net driving pressure difference is inversely related to the diffusive conductance. The net outward flux would continue until the bubble is completely resolved.

A bubble in tissue will likely be at a total pressure (P_t) somewhat different from barometric pressure (P_B). The mechanical stresses of tissue (ΔP_{tis}) will alter the total pressure, as will the pressure added by the surface forces (ΔP_S) of the bubble–liquid interface. As described in Chapter 3, a curved surface adds a total pressure component that is inversely proportional to the radius (R) of the surface and directly proportional to the surface tension (γ) as governed by LaPlace's Law.

$$\Delta P_S = \frac{2\gamma}{r} \qquad (11.3)$$

$$P_t = P_B + \Delta P_{tis} + \Delta P_S \qquad (11.4)$$

During the resolution process, the dynamics of diffusion are governed by the diffusion characteristics of the surrounding tissue. If the bubble is stationary within a large blood vessel, any convective flow will help carry away gas and thus enhance the rate of gas efflux. If the bubble is extravascular, diffusion distances will be greater and efflux will be slower. Any tissue perfusion will enhance the gas elimination. Smaller bubbles derive two types of benefit from the highly curved surface. First, the surface force along with the smaller radius of curvature will result in a greater ΔP_S elevating inert gas partial pressure within the bubble and increasing the outward diffusive driving force. Second, the curved surface results in a greater divergence of the gas flux lines and hence a more rapid drop in partial pressure with increasing distance from the surface, raising the partial pressure difference and the rate of gas efflux. In addition, the rate of absorption depends on local tissue perfusion rate. Increased perfusion enhances elimination of gas and results in more rapid resolution of the bubble.

The dynamics of resolution of bubbles have been studied in some detail. It is clear that the resolution dynamics depend on a great many factors, not the least of which are the geometry and perfusion of the surrounding tissue. The dynamics of bubble growth are considered to be symmetrical to bubble resolution for large bubbles; however, this is not true for small bubbles. The large ΔP_S of a very small, newly created bubble should raise internal pressure enough to make it difficult to diffuse gas into the bubble. Thus, it is difficult to imagine a set of circumstances permitting continued existence of very small (micro) bubbles.

Breath-Hold Diving

Diving without an air supply also has certain risks, owing to the combination of breath-holding and pressure change, which increases the potential for severe hypoxemia and blackout. The danger is encountered daily both by amateur divers and professional divers for shellfish and sponges in many countries around the world. As ambient total pressure increases during descent, there is a flux of N_2 from the alveolar gas into the blood and the development of a reversal of CO_2 flux from the alveolar gas to the blood. As ambient pressure decreases during ascent, the CO_2 and N_2 fluxes change, Pa_{CO_2} decreases, reducing ventilatory drive, so the diver is lulled into thinking there is adequate O_2 available. There is a substantial drop in the O_2 uptake by the blood because of the reduction in alveolar P_{O_2}. This pattern can be an even more serious threat if the diver hyperventilates before the dive; CO_2 is blown off, extending the period during the dive before build up of CO_2 provokes the urge to breathe, so that a more profound hypoxia and potential unconsciousness can occur near the end of the dive.

Inert Gas Narcosis

The high partial pressure of inert gases breathed at depth have an effect identical to that of anesthetic gases. The narcotic effect of inert gases is thought to relate to the solution of increased amounts of inert gas in cell membranes. The *Meyer-Overton hypothesis* states that the anesthetic potency of inert gases relates directly to the solubility in lipid. This effect is presumably manifested by a rise in membrane volume due to an increased number of dissolved inert gas molecules. Gases with higher lipid solubility require lower inert gas partial pressure to exhibit an anesthetic (or narcotic) effect. Narcotic potency may also relate, in part, to molecular weight, thermodynamic "activity," van der Waal's constants, and the formation of clathrates (lattice-like structures). For example, halothane has a high lipid solubility and high narcotic potency. The MAC (minimum alveolar concentration required for immobility in 50% of the subjects) for halothane is 0.0074 atm in humans, making it a suitable gas for anesthesia at sea level. Nitrogen has a low lipid solubility and narcotic potency. The MAC for N_2 is over 40 atm. At 1 atm it has no narcotic effect, but, as pressure increases over 3 atm, the narcotic effect of N_2 increases. At very high pressures, N_2 is an unsuitable breathing mixture because it causes narcosis. Therefore, alternative inert gases such as helium or hydrogen are used for dives to greater depths.

High Pressure Nervous Syndrome

With increases in absolute pressure, the central nervous system exhibits a general excitation (as opposed to the depression of inert gas narcosis) called *high pressure nervous syndrome* (HPNS). Symptoms include tremor of the hands, arms, or whole body; dizziness; nausea; and vomiting. HPNS has a "compression" (transient) component and a "hydrostatic pressure" (steady-state) component. The mechanism of HPNS is debated but may be due to the effects of pressure in reducing membrane volume. Experimental evidence shows that effects of inert gas narcosis (caused by membrane expansion by dissolved "inert gases") can be offset by increasing hydrostatic pressure. Presumably the opposite effects on the cell membrane result in a normal membrane volume. This observation has led to the use of trimix (5% to 10% N_2 in helium containing a small amount of O_2) to maintain appropriate inspired P_{O_2}, depending on depth). In this example, helium has a lesser narcotic potency, while the small amount of N_2 helps offset membrane compression by the hydrostatic pressure.

Oxygen Toxicity

As the diver breathes air at increasing pressures, the P_{O_2} eventually reaches levels high enough to be toxic to lung tissues and the central nervous system. The symptoms that develop depend on both P_{O_2} and duration of exposure. The pressure–duration relationship is shown in Figure 11.9. At low pressures (P_{O_2} between 0.5 and 2.2 atm), damage occurs primarily in the lungs. At higher pressures ($P_{O_2} >$ 2.6 atm), central nervous system symptoms occur before lung damage. For longer dives, O_2 toxicity can pose a serious problem unless care is taken to adjust the inspired O_2 fraction to maintain inspired P_{O_2} at less than 0.5 atm.

Carbon Monoxide Poisoning

Hyperbaric chambers are frequently used to treat carbon monoxide (CO) poisoning. CO, a by-product of combustion, reaches high levels in automobile exhaust, cigarette smoke, propane burners, and many other sources. CO competes with O_2 for the heme-binding sites on hemoglobin. Because of the high affinity of hemoglobin for CO, low levels of CO prevent the binding of O_2 by hemoglobin (see Chapter 6). Breathing O_2 at high pressure elevates the arterial P_{O_2} by a considerable amount ($P_{A_{O_2}}$ = 1300 mm Hg in a subject breathing 100% O_2 at 2.0 atm), which helps to drive off CO from the heme sites, increasing its rate of elimination. In addition, the markedly elevated P_{O_2} increases the amount of O_2 carried in physical solution (1.5 ml $\cdot$ dl^{-1} for every 500 mm Hg increase in $P_{A_{O_2}}$), enough to maintain O_2 delivery with only a limited amount of hemoglobin available for O_2 transport.

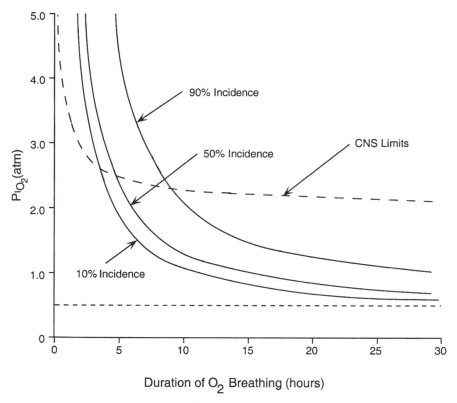

Duration of O_2 Breathing (hours)

Figure 11.9. Pulmonary (**solid lines**) and central nervous system (**long dashed lines**) O_2 tolerance curves for continuous exposures for normal human subjects. Horizontal **short dashed line** at 0.50 atm is the highest P_{IO_2} that can be breathed indefinitely without either central nervous system or pulmonary toxicity. (Adapted from Lambertsen CJ. Effects of hyperoxia on organs and their tissues. In: Lenfant C, executive editor. *Lung Biology in Health and Disease*, vol 8. Robin ED, editor. *Extrapulmonary Manifestations of Respiratory Disease*. New York: Marcel Dekker, 1978, pp 239–303.)

Further Reading

1. Bennett PB, Elliott DH. *The Physiology and Medicine of Diving and Compressed Air Work*. Baltimore: Williams & Wilkins, 1969.
2. Bisgard GE, Neubauer JA. Peripheral and central effects of hypoxia. In: Dempsey JA, Pack AI, editors. *Regulation of Breathing*, 2nd ed. New York: Marcel Dekker, 1995, pp 617–668.
3. Bove AA, Davis JC. *Diving Medicine*. Philadelphia: W B Saunders, 1990.
4. Dempsey JA, Forster HV. Mediation of ventilatory adaptations. *Physiol Rev* 62:262–346, 1982.

5. Dill DB. *Life, Heat, and Altitude*. Cambridge, MA: Harvard University Press, 1938, 211 pp.
6. Heath D, Williams DR. *High-Altitude Medicine and Pathology*. London: Butterworths, 1989, 352 pp.
7. Lenfant C, Sullivan K. Adaptation to high altitude. *N Engl J Med* 284:1298–1309, 1971.
8. Schoene RB, Hackett PH, Hornbein TF. High altitude. In: Murray JF, Nadel, JA, editors. *Textbook of Respiratory Medicine*, 2nd ed. Philadelphia: W B Saunders, 1994, pp 2062–2098.
9. Strauss RH. *Diving Medicine*. New York: Grune & Stratton, 1976.
10. Weil JV. Ventilatory control at high altitude. In: Cherniack NS, Widdicombe JG, editors. *Handbook of Physiology*, Section. 3, *The Respiratory System,* vol II, part 2, *Control of Breathing*. Bethesda, MD: American Physiological Society, 1986, pp 703–727.

Study Questions

11.1. Above approximately what altitude is permanent human habitation not feasible?

11.2. What is ventilatory acclimatization?

11.3. If an acclimatized subject is suddenly returned to sea level normoxic conditions, how will his or her ventilation change?

11.4. What adaptations take place in blood with long-term exposure to hypoxemia of altitude?

11.5. What is the most likely explanation for the increase in alveolar–arterial P_{O_2}?

11.6. If a 1 l volume of gas is taken from 33 fsw to 66 fsw, what will the new volume be?

11.7. Describe the washin and washout characteristics of inert gas in the human body within different tissues. Which tissues are the most likely for gas supersaturation and bubble formation?

11.8. Explain why bubbles in venous blood will always resolve.

11.9. How does absolute pressure and inert gas solution interact to affect behavior during deep dives?

11.10. Explain the advantages and disadvantages of using hyperbaric O_2 to treat CO poisoning.

12

Respiratory Physiology During Special States

In this chapter we examine three states that require the respiratory system to function differently than it does during normal quiet breathing: muscular exercise, with its increased metabolic demands that cause increased breathing; sleep; and the fetal and neonatal states, including the traumatic transition that occurs when *in utero* life becomes life outside the uterus.

Respiration During Exercise

The response to exercise requires coordination of the respiratory and cardiovascular systems. Exercise increases the demand for O_2 (expressed as increased $\dot{V}_{O_2}$ and the production of CO_2 (increased $\dot{V}_{CO_2}$) by increasing the activity and demands of skeletal muscle. To supply increased O_2 and remove excess CO_2, three primary physiological changes take place: (*1*) increased alveolar ventilation, (*2*) increased cardiac output, and (*3*) redistribution of cardiac output to enhance perfusion of exercising muscles.

Maximal O_2 uptake ($\dot{V}_{O_2}$ max) is determined by Fick's principle (Chapter 1):

$$\dot{V}_{O_2} \text{ max} = \dot{Q}(Ca_{O_2} - Cv_{O_2}) \tag{12.1}$$

Thus $\dot{V}_{O_2}$ max is determined by limitations in any of the three factors that comprise the right side of Fick's principle (Eq. 12.1). Each factor is governed primarily by a different system. The cardiovascular system determines cardiac output; the pulmonary exchange system regulates Ca_{O_2} and O_2 extraction and utilization by exercising muscle determine Cv_{O_2}. In this section, we discuss both cardiovascular and respiratory adaptations to exercise, but first we describe briefly the metabolic consequences of enhanced muscle metabolism during exercise.

Metabolic Effects

Increased muscle contraction during exercise requires the production of high-energy phosphate in the form of adenosine triphosphate (ATP). During mild to moderate exercise, ATP supply is increased by aerobic metabolism, that is, metabolism supported by O_2 consumption. Thus O_2 delivered by the respiratory and circulatory systems combines with metabolic substrates, such as carbohydrates and fatty acids, to form ATP. The main waste product of this metabolism is CO_2.

The amount of O_2 stored in the body is never great, and the amount of O_2 that can be delivered to the exercising muscles is limited. During *heavy exercise,* therefore, the O_2 supply to muscle cells is usually insufficient to meet the ATP demands of muscle contractions. When this occurs, anaerobic metabolism becomes an important source of ATP. Anaerobic metabolism is less efficient than aerobic metabolism because fewer ATP molecules are produced for each molecule of metabolic substrate consumed. Anaerobic metabolism involves lactic acid generation as a waste product, which is not as readily removed from the body as is CO_2. Thus, the ability of muscles to sustain anaerobic metabolism is more limited than their ability to sustain aerobic metabolism. As a consequence, anaerobic metabolism is more appropriate for short, intense periods of exercise (e.g., running 100 m) than for longer periods of exercise (e.g., running a marathon).

Figure 12.1 shows the progressive increase in $\dot{V}_{O_2}$ and $\dot{V}_{CO_2}$ with increasing degrees of exercise. The ratio of $\dot{V}_{CO_2} : \dot{V}_{O_2}$, R (the respiratory exchange ratio), remains constant up to a certain point (indicated by the dashed vertical line in Fig. 12.1). Above this point, because of the increased production of lactic acid and the bicarbonate buffering of the [H^+], the result is additional production of CO_2, which causes a further rise in $\dot{V}_{CO_2}$. This increases the ratio of $\dot{V}_{CO_2} : \dot{V}_{O_2}$ as additional CO_2 is exhaled.

Cardiovascular Responses

In ordinary active individuals, the cardiovascular system (mainly the heart) limits $\dot{V}_{O_2}$ max. While overall ventilation can increase by approximately 20-fold during maximal exercise, the heart increases its output by only about five times that of its normal resting output. The increase in cardiac output during exercise is due to large increases in heart rate and small increases in stroke volume. Figure 12.1 shows the progressive and linear increases in cardiac output that occur with increasing exercise intensity (O_2 consumption). Eventually cardiac output reaches a plateau. A number of mechanisms permit the level of exercise to rise higher than if cardiac output

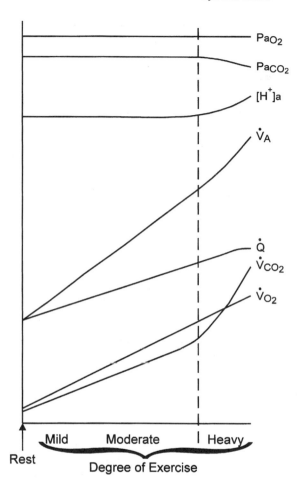

Figure 12.1. Schematic drawing illustrating the effects of increasing degrees of exercise on various respiratory and cardiovascular variables from a state of rest through heavy exercise. Vertical **dashed line** indicates the point above which, with increasing exercise intensity, the ratio of $\dot{V}_{CO_2}:\dot{V}_{O_2}$, R (the respiratory exchange ratio), increases.

were the sole determinant of exercise tolerance. Among these mechanisms is an increase in O_2 extraction from blood perfusing the exercising muscles, which causes venous P_{O_2} to fall.

Increased O_2 extraction is due in part to conditions in the exercising muscle that influence the oxygen–hemoglobin (O_2–Hb) dissociation curve. Increased temperature, decreased pH, and elevated P_{CO_2} of exercising muscle cause a rightward shift in the O_2–Hb dissociation curve. This shift promotes unloading of O_2 from blood to the exercising muscle (see Chapter 6) because the O_2 carrying capacity of blood is reduced at a given P_{O_2}, thereby increasing O_2 extraction.

During exercise, redistribution of blood flow is an important adaptive cardiovascular mechanism that increases perfusion of exercising muscles and skin. Overall, cardiac output becomes more effective in supplying exercising muscles with O_2 and metabolic substrates and in removing waste products. Redistribution is accomplished by vasoconstriction of vascular beds (including the splanchnic and renal beds) that are not directly involved in the exercise response and by vasodilatation of vascular beds within the exercising muscles. Increased perfusion of skin helps remove the excess body heat generated during exercise.

An interesting aspect of the cardiovascular response to exercise is the change in blood flow to respiratory muscles. During exercise, ventilation increases due to enhanced strength and rate of contractions of respiratory muscles. The blood flow to the respiratory muscles also increases during exercise. Under normal resting conditions, O_2 consumption by the respiratory muscles is about 5% of overall $\dot{V}_{O_2}$; during maximal exercise this can rise to 8% to 12% of $\dot{V}_{O_2}$. Certain mechanical properties of the respiratory system lead to this disproportionate intensification of breathing. As tidal volume increases, the lungs function on a less compliant portion of their pressure–volume relationship. Also at higher lung volumes, as seen during heavy exercise, the lungs and chest wall experience an inward recoil that requires increased work rate to expand the overall respiratory system during inspiration. Finally, with enhanced expiratory gas flows during exercise (see below), airway resistance is increased. These combined effects make the respiratory apparatus less energy efficient. Therefore, O_2 consumption by the respiratory muscles increases out of proportion to the overall increase in total $\dot{V}_{O_2}$.

Respiratory Responses

Respiratory Control in Exercise

Figure 12.1 shows that in humans during exercise below the point where R increases, arterial P_{O_2}, P_{CO_2} and $[H^+]$ remain unchanged from resting levels, but ventilation increases in proportion to the increase in $\dot{V}_{O_2}$ and $\dot{V}_{CO_2}$. The question is, because there is no arterial hypoxemia, hypercapnia, or acidemia, what provides the stimulus or drive for this additional ventilation? Possibilities are both neurally and humorally derived (blood-borne) stimuli. The distinguishing of neural from humoral stimuli is based on the changes that occur in ventilation at the beginning and end of exercise.

At the beginning of dynamic exercise, ventilation increases abruptly (Fig. 12.2), and then there is a progressive increase until ventilation reaches a steady-state level (Fig. 12.2). When exercise ceases, this sequence occurs in reverse, with ventilation diminishing abruptly at first and then gradually returning to resting levels. This description of the response to dynamic exercise is the basis for the *neurohumoral theory of ventilatory control in exercise*. According to this theory, the rapid rise in ventilation that occurs at the beginning of exercise is neural in origin, whereas the gradual increase observed as exercise progresses to a steady

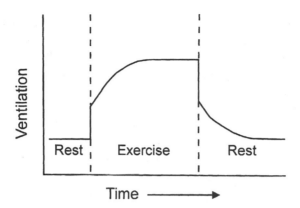

Figure 12.2. Time-dependent changes in ventilation observed at the initiation of exercise. Note abrupt increase in ventilation at the immediate onset of exercise, followed by a progressive increase as ventilation approaches its steady-state value. (Depiction derived from Dejours P. Control of respiration in muscular exercise. In: Fenn WO, Rahn H, editors. *Handbook of Physiology*, Section 3, *Respiration*, vol I. Washington, DC: American Physiological Society, 1964, pp 631–648.)

state is due to blood-borne stimuli. An increasing neural component, however, can contribute to the second phase.

Mechanisms that control breathing during exercise may arise from either the central or peripheral nervous system, or both. Feedforward and feedback control mechanisms, respectively, may be responsible for the exercise response. Feedforward control could be due to neural drive from the cerebral cortex, hypothalamus, or other central nervous system sites that may contribute to the increase in breathing during exercise. Although the exact mechanism by which the central nervous system stimulates breathing is unknown, animal experiments have demonstrated that electrical stimulation of sites in the hypothalamus can produce respiratory and cardiovascular responses that mimic those observed during exercise. Moreover, even in the absence of limb movements, as during fictive locomotion induced by central nervous system electrical stimulation (a condition in a *paralyzed* animal where rhythmic neural discharge in motor nerves to the limbs mimics those seen in exercise), phrenic nerve discharge increases as during normal exercise. These experiments support the hypothesis that an exercise-dependent *feedforward* drive to breathing is strictly central in origin. Such a feedforward neural mechanism may contribute, for example, to the rapid increase in breathing seen at the start of exercise.

Peripherally, groups I and II afferent fibers (the larger, myelinated afferent fibers from muscle spindles and tendon organs in exercising muscle) do not appear to influence the ventilatory response to exercise. In contrast, a small and limited contribution to ventilation during exercise may come from fiber groups III and IV. Group III myelinated fibers include muscle mechanoreceptors, whereas group IV unmyelinated fibers include nociceptors that can also be activated by various chemicals. Thus during exercise, muscle contraction and metabolite production can activate these receptors and thereby contribute, in part, to the increased ventilation.

Blood-borne factors can play a role in the *feedback* response to exercise. The constancy of P_{O_2}, P_{CO_2} and $[H^+]$ at mild to moderate levels of exercise has been mentioned previously. Figure 12.3 illustrates the relationship between $\dot{V}_A$ and P_{ACO_2}. At a constant value of $\dot{V}_{CO_2}$, the two variables, $\dot{V}_A$ and P_{ACO_2}, are inversely related (see Chapter 4). If $\dot{V}_{CO_2}$ is raised to a higher level, as during mild or moderate steady-state exercise, then $\dot{V}_A$ and P_{ACO_2} are also related via another hyperbolic

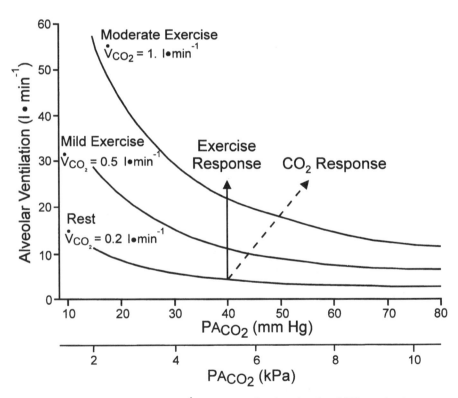

Figure 12.3. Relationships between $\dot{V}_A$ and P_{ACO_2} for three levels of CO_2 production: at rest and during mild and moderate exercise. **Dashed line** indicates the ventilatory response to increasing P_{ACO_2} (ventilatory control line). **Solid vertical line** indicates the ventilatory response (isocapnic) observed with increasing degrees of exercise. Note that the discrepancy between solid and dashed lines indicates that the ventilation observed during exercise is not explained by the ventilatory control system's response to the increase in P_{ACO_2}.

relationship that lies above the original one. In mild or moderate exercise $P_{A_{CO_2}}$ does not change, yet $\dot{V}_A$ increases. Therefore, a factor other than $P_{A_{CO_2}}$ must account for the increase in $\dot{V}_A$. If $P_{A_{CO_2}}$ were the cause of the increased $\dot{V}_A$ during exercise, then $P_{A_{CO_2}}$ would have to rise along the line defining the CO_2 control system response (the subject's ventilatory response to an increase in Pa_{CO_2}), which does not happen (see Chapter 9). One way to explain this apparent dilemma is that new receptors or new properties of known receptors may cause respiration to increase during exercise. Increased sensory input from the carotid chemoreceptors and venous CO_2 flow receptors are two possibilities. In the first case it is known that, with an increase in tidal volume, there are increased peak to peak changes in arterial P_{CO_2} and [H^+] that can contribute to an increased breathing rate if the carotid bodies are sensitive to rate of change as well as to mean levels of these variables. Another possibility is the existence of a receptor that is sensitive to CO_2 flow coming back to the lungs via the venous return. No definitive evidence has been found for any of the sensory mechanisms that may have a role in the steady-state exercise response.

Respiratory drive during heavy exercise may involve increased sensory inputs to the central nervous system that arise from increases in plasma levels of [H^+], norepinephrine, and K^+ that occur under this condition. Increased arterial blood [H^+], due to lactic acid production by muscles, may be sensed by the carotid chemoreceptors and thus may contribute to increased ventilation. Norepinephrine concentration is elevated by sympathetic stimulation and, along with the elevated plasma K^+ produced by the exercising muscle, it may stimulate ventilation. The factor or factors responsible for the exercise hyperpnea remain controversial.

In summary, increased breathing during mild to moderate exercise, in the presence of constant steady-state arterial blood gas measurements (P_{O_2}, P_{CO_2} and [H^+]), requires some other sensory input or central nervous system mechanism(s) to be responsible for increased breathing. During heavy exercise, various blood-borne factors, including [H^+], norepinephrine, and K^+, may be important in producing the additional increase in ventilation.

Pulmonary System Adaptations During Exercise

In addition to control mechanism changes during exercise, other important adaptive alterations occur within the pulmonary system. For example, Figure 12.4 shows that at increased levels of exercise there are decreases in the fraction of the volume of each breath that goes to wasted ventilation (the physiological dead space). At rest, the V_D: V_T ratio is normally about 1:3; it drops to about 1:10 during high levels of exercise when V_T is increased. Therefore, normal $\dot{V}_A$ levels will rise from about two-thirds to about nine-tenths of total ventilation during heavy exercise, resulting in more efficient gas exchange in the lungs. The primary reason for the

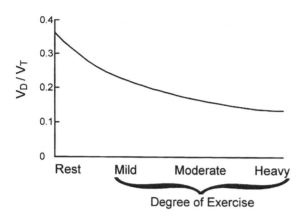

Figure 12.4. Effect of increasing degrees of exercise on the physiologic dead space/tidal volume ratio (V_D/V_T).

fall in the V_D: V_T ratio with exercise is due to the small change in V_D in the face of large increases in V_T in exercise. Why does V_D change so little? Recall (Chapter 4) that physiologic dead space is the sum of the anatomic and alveolar dead spaces. The anatomical dead space will increase somewhat as the airways expand at the larger lung volumes seen in exercise. In contrast, the alveolar dead space will decrease because there will be increased perfusion of previously closed pulmonary capillaries (recruitment) and increased distention of other pulmonary capillaries as cardiac output rises during exercise. Furthermore, pulmonary arterial pressure will rise only modestly due to the recruitment and distension of pulmonary capillaries despite the large increase in cardiac output during exercise.

The mechanical responses of the lungs and chest wall are another important feature of the exercise response. An important question is, do the mechanical properties of the respiratory system limit the required ventilation? This is generally not the case. With progressively increasing levels of exercise, an individual utilizes greater amounts of both inspiratory *and* expiratory reserve volumes to generate the enhanced ventilation. It has been pointed out that the respiratory gas flow–lung volume loops (see Chapter 3) observed in an untrained individual become larger as $\dot{V}_{O_2}$ increases (Fig. 12.5), but in a normally active individual these loops rarely reach the flow–lung volume loop obtained by maximum voluntary ventilation. Thus normal, untrained individuals, whose cardiovascular systems usually limit their exercise responses, have a mechanical reserve within the maximum voluntary respiratory gas flow–lung volume loop. In contrast, some highly trained young athletes and older individuals exhibit maximal expiratory flows during much of the expired phase of the respiratory cycle, which reduces the usual degree of hyperventilation seen at elevated levels of exercise.

During exercise there is an increase in pulmonary capillary blood volume. In

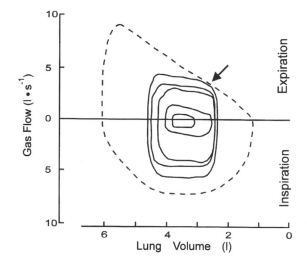

Figure 12.5. Respiratory gas flow–lung volume loops observed in a young untrained adult. **Dashed line** indicates the maximal voluntary ventilation loop obtained with the subject at rest. Progressively increasing loops (**solid lines**) are obtained, starting with the subject at rest (**innermost loop**) and at progressively increasing levels of exercise until the **outermost solid-line loop** is at the subject's $\dot{V}_{O_2}$ max. (Adapted from Dempsey JA et al. Adaptations and limitations in the pulmonary system during exercise. *Chest* [Suppl] 97: 81S–87S, 1990.)

normally active individuals this increased pulmonary capillary blood volume during high pulmonary blood flow will lessen the reduction in pulmonary capillary red cell transit time. This mechanism helps to prevent arterial hypoxemia. Nevertheless, with increasing $\dot{V}_{O_2}$, there is a progressive increase in the alveolar–arterial P_{O_2} difference. In normally active individuals at $\dot{V}_{O_2}$ max this difference may approach 20 to 30 mm Hg because hyperventilation causes alveolar P_{O_2} to rise (see Fig. 12.1) while the decrease in arterial P_{O_2} is insignificant.

A major reason why arterial P_{O_2} does not rise as alveolar P_{O_2} rises appears to be the delivery of markedly desaturated venous blood traversing the normal anatomical shunt into the arterial side of the circulation. The increased desaturation of venous blood stems from the increased O_2 extraction in the exercising muscles. Another reason for the increased alveolar–arterial P_{O_2} difference is the increased $\dot{V}/\dot{Q}$ dispersion. This occurs even though the overall $\dot{V}/\dot{Q}$ rises markedly during heavy exercise due to the disproportionate increase in $\dot{V}_A$ compared with the increase in $\dot{Q}$ (see Fig. 12.1).

During heavy exercise a small number of highly trained elite athletes exhibit marked disequilibrium between alveolar and end-pulmonary capillary P_{O_2}, which can result in arterial hypoxemia. This disequilibrium results from the enhanced capability through training of the cardiovascular system to increase cardiac output and, hence, pulmonary blood flow to very high levels. This training does not apparently increase the gas-exchanging capabilities of the lungs per se. The arterial

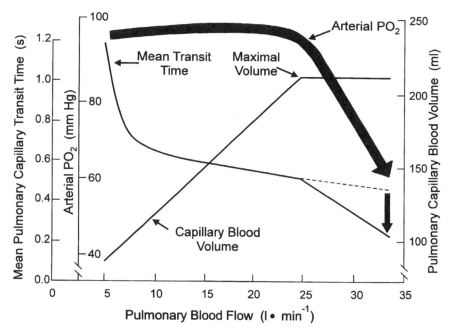

Figure 12.6. Reductions in mean pulmonary capillary red cell transit time after maximal pulmonary capillary blood volume is reached can cause marked arterial hypoxemia. This schema may explain why some highly trained athletes exhibit marked arterial hypoxemia during severe exercise. (Rowell LB. *Human Cardiovascular Control*, ch. 9. New York: Oxford University Press, 1993, pp 326–370.)

hypoxemia in these athletes can limit $\dot{V}_{O_2}$ max. Most likely, the observed arterial hypoxemia is explained by the presence of diffusion disequilibrium between alveolar and end-pulmonary capillary P_{O_2}. These special individuals have very high cardiac outputs when exercising intensely. Perhaps there is insufficient time to achieve equilibrium between alveolar gas and capillary blood as the transit time of red blood cells within the pulmonary capillaries is decreased. Figure 12.6 illustrates an example of this phenomenon and shows that, at a high level of pulmonary blood flow, the pulmonary blood volume cannot expand further; at this point pulmonary capillary transit time markedly decreases, resulting in alveolar to end-capillary disequilibrium and arterial hypoxemia.

Respiration During Sleep

Humans spend about 30% of their lives sleeping; thus it is of interest to know how respiration is altered during sleep. Sleep is not homogeneous; it has been broadly divided into two distinct states. During sleep humans cycle between these two states with an average overall period of 90 minutes. One state is called *non-rapid eye movement* (NREM) or *quiet sleep;* it has four substages. The deepest and last two stages, 3 and 4, are called *slow-wave sleep.* NREM is characterized by varying degrees of large amplitude electroencephalographic activity and the presence of tonic electromyographic activity. The other major sleep state is *rapid eye movement* (REM) *sleep,* sometimes called *active* or *desynchronized sleep.* REM is characterized by bursts of REMs, a desynchronized electroencephalographic activity, dreaming, and a loss of muscle tone.

The pattern of breathing in NREM is distinguished by its regularity. During NREM a decrease in $\dot{V}_A$ and an increase in arterial P_{CO_2} occur; thus there is a reduction in ventilation with respect to metabolism even though $\dot{V}_{CO_2}$ decreases from awake-state values. Figure 12.7 shows the progressive drop in overall ventilation that occurs from the awake state through stages 2 and 4 of NREM sleep. Compared with wakefulness, the ventilatory response to inhaled CO_2 is reduced in NREM sleep, and the ventilatory response to isocapnic hypoxia in NREM sleep is also reduced.

During REM sleep, respiration can be irregular. Figure 12.7 shows that in REM overall $\dot{V}$ tends to be somewhat higher than in NREM, but is still somewhat reduced from the awake state. In REM respiratory muscle activity is markedly altered from that observed in either the awake state or in NREM. Tonic intercostal muscle activity is partly abolished during REM, and its rhythmic activity is substantially reduced. Phasic diaphragmatic activity compensates for the loss of intercostal activity in REM.

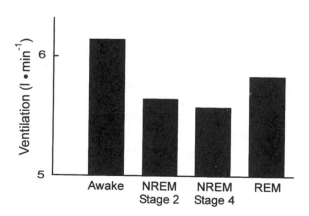

Figure 12.7. Changes in overall ventilation versus sleep state. Mean data from normal subjects are shown. Overall ventilation was significantly altered with state; it was greatest during the awake state, lowest during NREM sleep stage 4, and in between during REM sleep. (Adapted from Tabachnik E et al. Changes in ventilation and chest wall mechanics during sleep in normal adolescents. *J Appl Physiol* 51:557–564, 1981.)

Arterial oxygenation decreases during REM. Arterial P_{CO_2} values during REM are similar to those measured during NREM sleep, and the ventilatory response to inhaled CO_2 is variable but has been found to range from that observed in NREM to being markedly diminished. Also, in REM there are small decreases in the ventilatory response to hypoxia compared with that observed in NREM sleep.

Certain pathophysiological conditions are associated with sleep. One such condition, sleep apnea, is defined as the cessation of airflow at the mouth and nostrils for a period of at least 10 seconds and this occurring at least 15 times per hour. Sleep apnea can be either obstructive or central or both (the last termed *mixed apnea*). Obstructive sleep apnea is distinguished by a closure of the upper airway at the level of the oropharynx despite the presence of persistent respiratory efforts by the diaphragm and intercostals, the main muscles involved in breathing. Central apnea occurs when rhythmic activity in all respiratory muscles stops and a cessation of airflow follows due to failure of the central respiratory rhythm-generating mechanism. Apnea can also arise from a combination of both obstructive and central events.

Apnea ends with the subject either awakening or passing to a less-deep stage of sleep. The reasons for arousal are complex, probably involving stimulation of chemosensors due to hypoxemia and hypercapnia caused by the apnea. Also, in obstructive sleep apnea, mechanical factors associated with the pressure forces across the airways may play a role in terminating the apnea. There are a number of clinical features associated with sleep apnea; left heart failure, pulmonary hypertension and its associated right heart failure, systemic hypertension, and profound daytime sleepiness.

Figure 12.8 shows the primary sites of obstruction in the oropharyngeal airway that are found in patients with obstructive sleep apnea. Two sites predominate, one at the level of the soft palate (retropalatal) and the other at the base of the tongue (retroglossal). Airway closure can depend on anatomical factors such as variations in size of the upper airway opening and the balance of forces directed to the upper airways as gas goes in and out of the airway (Bernoulli effect). Also, sleep state can profoundly influence airway closure. For example, Figure 12.9 shows that during the rapid eye movements occurring in REM sleep, there is a marked loss of tonic and inspiratory phase–linked activity in the genioglossus muscle, the muscle that causes tongue protrusion. This loss in activity coincides with a profound reduction in tidal volume, pointing to the possible role of sleep state and loss of tone in the tongue muscle as potential causes of some forms of obstructive sleep apnea. A current treatment for obstructive sleep apnea is nasal continuous positive airway pressure (CPAP). Nasal CPAP involves blowing air through the nose into the upper airway, thereby effectively "splinting" the upper airway and preventing airway collapse.

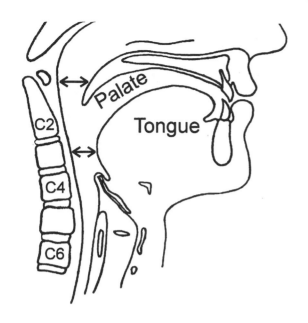

Figure 12.8. Primary locations of upper airway obstruction in patients with obstructive sleep apnea. **Arrows** indicate the location of sites of obstruction, just behind the soft palate (retropalatal) and at the base of the tongue (retroglossal). (Adapted from Chaban R et al. Site of upper airway obstruction in patients with idiopathic obstructive sleep apnea. *Laryngoscope* 98:641–647, 1988.)

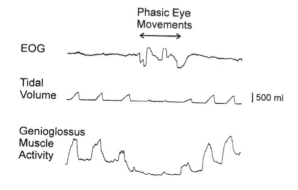

Figure 12.9. Loss of rhythmic and tonic genioglossus muscle activity and near-abolition of tidal volume during phasic eye movements of REM sleep in a normal subject. Eye movements indicated by electro-oculogram (EOG, **top trace**). (Adapted from Wiegand L et al. Changes in upper airway muscle activation and ventilation during phasic REM sleep in normal men. *J Appl Physiol* 71:488–497, 1991.)

Respiration in the Fetus and Neonate

The fetus is fully immersed in amniotic fluid within the uterus. Consequently, fetal lungs do not function as blood gas exchangers. The placenta enables gas exchange to occur between maternal and fetal blood. Just before birth, approximately one-half of the cardiac output passes to the placenta for gas exchange. At birth, with clamping, tying, and cutting of the umbilical cord, the placenta is lost as a gas exchanger when it is separated from the uterus. At this point the newborn's lungs and internal circulatory system must be ready to undertake the critical function of gas exchange in a very short period of time if the newborn is to survive. This section focuses on three key questions about the transition from *in utero* life: (*1*) how does fetal and neonatal respiratory gas exchange occur, (*2*) how do the lungs grow and develop during this time, and (*3*) how does the control of breathing develop?

Respiratory Gas Exchange

The fetal circulatory system is adapted to the placenta, not the lungs, for gas exchange. Figure 12.10 illustrates the three key elements of the fetal circulatory system that channel oxygenated blood from the placenta into the aorta for distribution to the vital organs: the ductus arteriosus, the foramen ovale, and the ductus venosus. These three structures close after birth, creating an adult-like circulatory system in the early neonatal period.

In the fetus only a small portion of the blood leaving the right heart passes to the fetal lungs; most blood enters the ductus arteriosus, which shunts blood directly into the aorta, bypassing the lungs and left heart. This shunt occurs because *in utero* pulmonary vascular resistance is quite high, in part because of reduced levels of P_{O_2} in the lungs, causing pulmonary hypoxic vasoconstriction. After birth, pulmonary vascular resistance and pulmonary arterial pressure decrease (Figure 12.11), causing flow to reverse in the ductus arteriosus as the pulmonary arterial pressure drops. During the immediate postnatal period, the ductus arteriosus closes, and blood flow through this structure declines.

The presence of the foramen ovale enables blood to pass from the inferior vena cava directly into the left atrium (Fig. 12.10). Blood returning from the lower limbs and gut, as well as the placenta, flows into the left side of the heart, bypassing the pulmonary circulation. *In utero*, less than 10% of cardiac output perfuses the lungs due to the combined effects of the foramen ovale and ductus arteriosus. After birth the lungs receive most of the cardiac output. Another consequence of these two structures is that both sides of the fetal heart appear to function in parallel, both pumping blood from veins to the aorta. The filling and ejection pressures and right and left heart capacities are similar in the fetal heart.

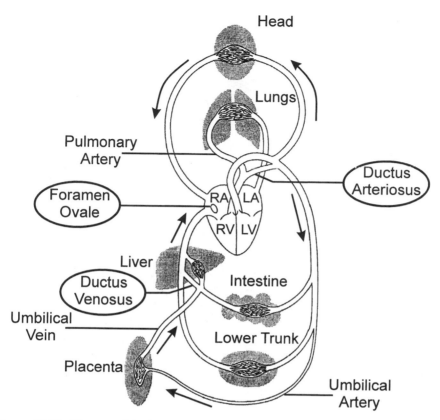

Figure 12.10. Diagram of the human fetal circulation. LA, RA, left and right atrium, respectively; LV, RV, left and right ventricle, respectively. (Adapted from Rudolph AM, Heymann MA. The circulation of the fetus in utero. *Circ Res* 21:163–184, 1967.)

The ductus venosus enables a large proportion of blood returned to the fetus in the umbilical vein to go directly into the inferior vena cava, bypassing the liver. Unlike other venous blood being returned to the fetal heart, this blood has a high P_{O_2} and a low P_{CO_2} following gas exchange with maternal blood in the placenta.

In addition to circulatory mechanisms that permit gas exchange to occur in the placenta, there are other important differences in the fetal gas transport system. For example, the type of hemoglobin found in fetal blood has a much greater affinity for O_2 than that of adult blood. As discussed in Chapter 6, adult hemoglobin (HbA) is composed of α- and β-chains. In contrast, in fetal hemoglobin (HbF), γ-chains replace β-chains. The P_{50} of fetal blood is much lower than that of adult blood (19 compared with 27 mm Hg, respectively).

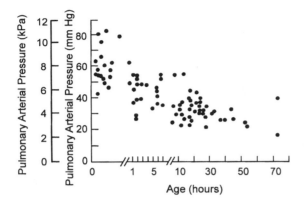

Figure 12.11. Pulmonary arterial pressure as a function of age from birth in normal human infants. (Adapted from Dawes GS. *Foetal and Neonatal Physiology.* Chicago: Year Book Medical Publishers, 1968, p 167.)

The physiological consequence of the higher O_2 affinity of fetal blood compared with adult blood is elevated O_2 carrying capacity at the same P_{O_2} level (Fig. 12.12). The increased hematocrit of fetal blood also contributes to this increased capacity. At birth, Hb concentration is about 18 gm $\cdot$ dl^{-1}, whereas it is 15 gm $\cdot$ dl^{-1} in the normal adult. Thus fetal blood has an O_2 content of approximately 24 ml $\cdot$ dl^{-1} when saturated, whereas adult values are about 20 ml $\cdot$ dl^{-1} under the same condition. Table 12.1 shows fetal arterial P_{O_2} (in the umbilical vein) to be about one-fourth that of the mother, even though the O_2 content of fetal arterial blood is not much lower than that of the mother's arterial blood (Fig. 12.12). Thus within the placenta, fetal blood can pick up large quantities of O_2. Table 12.1 also shows that fetal blood traversing across the placenta increases pH levels and reduces P_{CO_2} (Bohr effect), which contributes to the O_2 transfer from maternal to fetal blood. Figure 12.12 shows that the O_2 equilibrium curve is steeper for fetal than for adult (maternal) blood—an advantage in fetal tissues where small reductions in P_{O_2} across

Table 12.1. Average Blood Gas Values in Mother and Fetus*

	MATERNAL ARTERIAL BLOOD	FETAL UMBILICAL VEIN	FETAL UMBILICAL ARTERY
P_{O_2}, mm Hg	97	29	18
P_{CO_2}, mm Hg	26	37	41
pH	7.48	7.31	7.26

* Ten patients undergoing cesarean delivery at term.

Data from: Spackman T, Fuchs F, Assali NS. Acid–base status of the fetus in human pregnancy. *Obstet Gynecol* 22: 785–791, 1963.

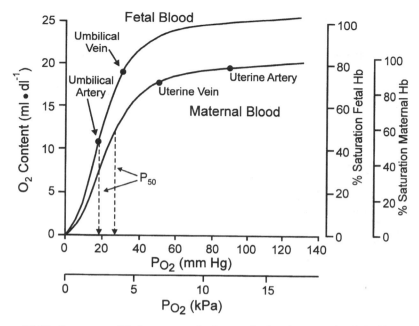

Figure 12.12. Oxygen equilibrium curves for human fetal and maternal (adult) blood. Also indicated are the O_2 contents and P_{O_2} values of the umbilical artery and vein and the uterine artery and vein as well as the P_{50} and the percent saturation of fetal and maternal hemoglobin.

the capillaries results in the delivery of large amounts of O_2 to these tissues. These differences in fetal blood and circulation compared with the adult enable the fetus to survive in the *in utero* hypoxic environment.

Lung Growth and Development

Even though the lungs do not function as gas exchangers *in utero*, lung growth and development are essential to prepare the fetus for an air-breathing life after birth. Structural growth and development occur throughout the *in utero* period and extend into postnatal life. Development occurs in three chronological phases: embryonic, fetal, and postnatal. In humans the embryonic phase occurs during the first 5 to 7 weeks following fertilization. At about day 26 the lung appears as a bud from the esophagus, and by day 37 airways extending to the lobar bronchi are formed. Several important aspects of lung development during the fetal and postnatal periods have been summarized by Reid in her *Laws of Development of the Human Lung:*

1. The bronchial tree is developed by the 16th week of intrauterine life.
2. Alveoli continue to develop after birth, increasing in number until the age of 8 years and in size until growth of the chest wall is complete.
3. Blood vessels are remodeled and increase in number, certainly while new alveoli are forming and probably until the growth of the chest is complete.

Figure 12.13 shows the development of the intrasegmental bronchial airway tree during fetal and postnatal periods. During the fetal period, lung development can be divided into three chronological stages: pseudoglandular, canalicular, and saccular stages. During the pseudoglandular stage, the lung has a gland-like appearance, the bronchial divisions are established, but respiration is not possible because the branching airways have blind ends. The canalicular stage is characterized by (*1*) development of the respiratory acinus (this is the terminal respiratory unit consisting of respiratory bronchioles, alveolar ducts and alveoli), (*2*) differentiation of the pulmonary epithelium, and (*3*) development of the typical blood–

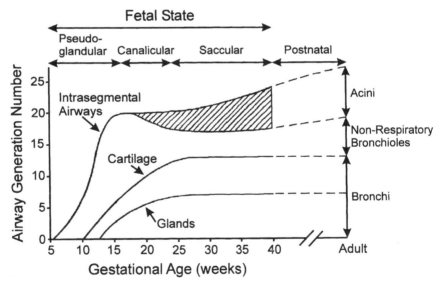

Figure 12.13. Development of the intrasegmental bronchial tree. Upper line indicates the development of the intrasegmental airways that start at about fetal age 6 weeks. Shaded area is the respiratory zone of the bronchial tree, including respiratory bronchioles, alveolar ducts, and alveoli. Also shown is the development of cartilage and glands in the bronchial tree. Airway generation number fitted to the dichotomous branching scheme of Weibel. (Adapted from Bucher U, Reid L. Development of the intrasegmental bronchial tree: The pattern of branching and development of cartilage at various stages of intra-uterine life. *Thorax* 16: 207–218, 1961.)

gas barrier during this period as the capillaries invade the epithelium (saccular stage). The saccular stage is characterized by further development of the alveolar duct system, airway growth (notably those airways peripheral to the terminal bronchioles), development of a thin blood–gas barrier, and progressive maturation of the lung surfactant system. After birth the alveoli continue to develop up to about 8 years of age. At birth there are about 20×10^6 alveoli, and at 8 years of age there are about 300×10^6 alveoli.

The development of the lung surfactant system has important clinical implications. Studies of fetal lambs have shown that lamellar bodies of the alveolar type II cells, those that secrete surfactant, appear approximately 5 days before the detectable presence of surfactant. In lambs surfactant is first detected at about 125 days' gestation; birth occurs at 147 days. In humans the lungs start to contain surfactant at about 210 days' gestation, while birth is at 280 days. Figure 12.14 shows the functional consequences of maturation of the surfactant-secreting system in the lungs.

The pressure–volume curves of the lungs of a fetal lamb at 140 days' gestation (95% of term), a point during fetal development when surfactant is in the alveolar lining liquid, are shown in Figure 12.14A1. The solid curve reveals that the first inflation requires about 18 cm H_2O to instill a significant amount of air into the

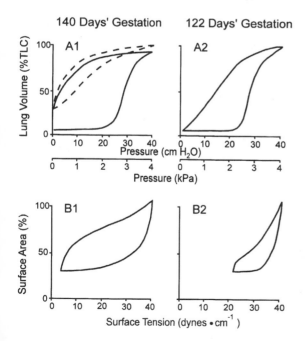

Figure 12.14. Pressure–volume curves (**A**) and surface tension versus area (**B**) derived from mature (**left side**) and immature (**right side**) fetal lambs. A1 and B1 are from a lamb of 140 days' gestation, and A2 and B2 are from a lamb of 122 days' gestation. See text for a detailed description. (Adapted from Reynolds EOR, Strang LB. Alveolar surface properties of the lung in the new-born. *Br Med Bull* 22:79–83, 1966.)

lungs (called the *opening pressure*); with additional pressure, the lungs easily fill to capacity. The deflation curve is separated from the inflation curve, exhibiting hysteresis. At zero pressure the lungs retain about 25% of their total volume. The second inflation (dashed line) shows that no opening pressure is required for inflation of the lungs to occur; at the opening pressure of the first breath, the lungs are now filled to about 80% of total volume. Figure 12.14A2 shows that the pressure–volume curves of a fetal lamb at 122 days' gestation (83% of term) are somewhat different from those of the older fetus. Recall that surfactant is not detected in the fetal lamb lungs at this gestational age. Although the initial inflation curve is similar to that seen in the older fetus, the lungs collapse at zero pressure on deflation. The inflation and deflation curves for the second breath are the same as for the first. Large opening pressures are still required, and at the end of deflation the lungs collapse.

The differences in these pressure–volume curves at the two gestational ages can be interpreted by examining the surface-tension properties of the alveolar lining liquid layer. Figure 12.14B1 and B2 shows the surface tension of the lining liquid layer taken from lung extracts from these two fetal lambs. Figure 12.14B1 reveals marked decreases in surface tension with reductions in surface area (lung volume) in the more mature fetus, as shown previously for lung surfactant from adult lungs (see Fig. 3–6). This property minimizes the tendency for the alveoli to collapse due to the surface tension forces at the liquid–air interface. Also as shown in Figure 12.14B1, the presence of a large degree of hysteresis is similar to that seen for normal lung surfactant from adult lungs. In contrast, the surface tension in the younger fetus is much higher during compression of the surface film, and the degree of hysteresis is markedly reduced (Figure 12.14B2). Therefore the higher surface tension in the younger fetus favors alveoli collapse on deflation. In the less mature fetus, the lungs must reopen for each breath, and the work of breathing is therefore considerably greater than in the older fetus. The clinical implications of this developmental regulation of surfactant production became apparent when Avery and Mead in 1959 observed that infants dying of respiratory distress syndrome (IRDS) lacked surfactant in their lungs. Recent evidence indicates that delivery of exogenous surfactant to the lungs of premature infants lowers the incidence of respiratory distress syndrome.

Development of the Control of Breathing

The transition from *in utero* life is one of the greatest challenges that the organism must face. One important aspect of the transition is breathing, which must go from episodic, irregular, and ineffectual to regular, rhythmic, and effectual respiratory movements. A number of studies have shown that the *in utero* fetus makes frequent, shallow, irregular respiratory movements during the last half of gestation. Although the physiological basis for the first breath at birth is unknown, many possible factors are apparent, including the large number of sensory stimuli that bombard the newborn. Both external stimuli (such as light, sound, touch, added gravitational forces, odors, and reduced external temperature) and internal stimuli (including reductions in blood P_{O_2} and pH and elevations in P_{CO_2} that activate central and peripheral arterial chemosensors) are present.

The respiratory response to hypoxemia in the fetus is different from that in the adult. Hypoxemia markedly diminishes fetal breathing movements. This may be an appropriate adaptation for the fetus because it does not rely on respiratory movements for gas exchange, and the inhibition of respiratory movements due to hypoxemia reduces O_2 demand by the fetus. During the immediate postnatal period, the ventilatory response to hypoxemia exhibits a biphasic structure. Initially there is increased ventilation, and then ventilation returns to prehypoxemic levels or drops below them. About 1 week after delivery at term, the newborn has a sustained ventilatory response to hypoxemia, that is, an adult-like response pattern. The mechanisms for this biphasic response are not understood but may be due to mechanical factors involving the lungs and chest wall, delayed maturation of respiratory-related neurotransmitter systems in the brain, and postnatal maturation of the peripheral arterial chemosensor system. In contrast to the hypoxemic response, elevation in fetal arterial P_{CO_2} causes the fetus to increase its breathing movements. Infants born preterm show diminished ventilatory sensitivity to CO_2, unlike infants born at term, who have an adult-like CO_2 response.

Further Reading

A. Response to Exercise

1. Dempsey JA, Forster HV, Ainsworth DM. Regulation of hyperpnea, hyperventilation, and respiratory muscle recruitment during exercise. In: Dempsey JA, Pack AI, editors. *Regulation of Breathing*, 2nd ed. New York: Marcel Dekker, 1995, pp 1065–1134.
2. Eldridge FL, Millhorn DE, Waldrop TG. Stimulation by central command of locomotion, respiration and circulation during exercise. *Respir Physiol* 59:313–337, 1985.
3. Murray JF. *The Normal Lung,* 2nd ed,. Philadelphia: WB Saunders, 1986, pp 261–282.
4. Paterson DJ. Potassium and ventilation in exercise. *J Appl Physiol* 72:811–820, 1992.
5. Rowell LB. *Human Cardiovascular Control.* New York: Oxford University Press, 1993, pp 326–370.
6. Whipp BJ. Breathing during exercise. In: Fishman AP, editor. *Pulmonary Diseases and Disorders,* 3rd ed. New York: McGraw-Hill, 1998, pp 229–241.

B. Response to Sleep

1. Hudgel DW. Mechanisms of obstructive sleep apnea. *Chest* 101:541–549, 1992.
2. Pack AI, Kubin L, Davies RO. Changes in the cardiovascular system during sleep. In:

Fishman AP, editor. *Pulmonary Diseases and Disorders*, 3rd ed. New York: McGraw-Hill, 1998, pp 1607–1615.

3. Phillipson EA. Sleep disorders. In: Murray JF, Nadel JA, editors. *Textbook of Respiratory Medicine*, 2nd ed. Philadelphia: WB Saunders, 1994, pp 2301–2324.

4. Saunders NA, Sullivan CE, editors. *Sleep and Breathing*, 2nd ed, vol 71, *Lung Biology in Health and Disease*. New York: Marcel Dekker, 1994.

5. Schwab RJ, Goldberg AN, Pack AI. Sleep apnea syndromes. In: Fishman AP, editor. *Pulmonary Diseases and Disorders,* 3rd ed. New York: McGraw-Hill, 1998, pp 1617–1637.

C. Fetal and Neonatal Respiration

1. Avery ME, Mead J. Surface properties in relation to atelectasis and hyaline membrane disease. *JAMA Dis Child* 97:517–523, 1959.

2. Bryan AC, Bowes G, Maloney JE. Control of breathing in the fetus and the newborn. In: Cherniack NS, Widdicombe JG, editors. *Handbook of Physiology*, Section 3, *The Respiratory System*, vol II, part 2, *Control of Breathing*. Bethesda, MD: American Physiological Society, 1986, pp 621–647.

3. Burri PH. Development and growth of the lung. In: Fishman AP, editor. *Pulmonary Diseases and Disorders*, 3rd ed. New York: McGraw-Hill, 1998, pp 91–105.

4. Dawes GS. *Foetal and Neonatal Physiology*. Chicago: Year Book Medical Publishers, 1968.

5. Haddad GG, Farber JP, editors. *Developmental Neurobiology of Breathing*, vol 53, *Lung Biology in Health and Disease*. New York: Marcel Dekker, 1991.

6. Jansen AH, Chernick V. Fetal breathing and development of control of breathing. *J Appl Physiol* 70:1431–1446, 1991.

7. Reid L. The embryology of the lung. In: De Reuck AVS, Porter R, editors. *Development of the Lung*. Boston: Little, Brown and Co, 1967, pp 109–124.

8. Scarpelli EM, editor. *Pulmonary Physiology: Fetus, Newborn Child and Adolescent,* 2nd ed. Philadelphia: Lea & Febiger, 1990.

Study Questions

12.1. Name three factors that can limit maximal O_2 consumption during exercise.

12.2. In mild to moderate exercise, describe the changes that occur in arterial P_{O_2}, P_{CO_2}, and pH from their levels during resting control conditions.

12.3. What substances in plasma may contribute to the increased respiratory drive during heavy exercise?

12.4. During heavy exercise a small number of highly trained elite athletes exhibit marked disequilibrium between alveolar and end-pulmonary capillary P_{O_2} that can result in arterial hypoxemia. What is the mechanism for this disequilibrium?

12.5. Describe the two main sleep states.

12.6. Describe the changes that occur in ventilation during sleep compared with ventilation in the awake state.

12.7. Describe what is meant by obstructive sleep apnea and what factors can influence this pathology.

12.8. Name the three structures that channel oxygenated blood from the placenta to the aorta of the fetus.

12.9. How do HbA and HbF differ structurally and functionally?

12.10. The development of the lung surfactant system has important clinical implications. Describe the differences in the pressure–volume curves of the lungs lacking a mature pulmonary surfactant system from those with one.

13

Acid–Base Regulation

The concentration of H^+ ($[H^+]$) in various compartments of the body is critical to homeostasis. Because the respiratory system has a key role in H^+ regulation through CO_2 excretion by the lungs, we need to understand acid-base regulation. In addition to the lungs, the kidneys are also important in H^+ regulation. In this chapter we first develop some basic concepts of acid–base chemistry. Later we apply these to the understanding of acid–base regulation in the body.

We focus on H^+ in arterial blood, where its concentration deviates little from its normal value of 40×10^{-9} equivalents $\cdot$ l^{-1} (40 nanoEq $\cdot$ l^{-1} or nEq $\cdot$ l^{-1}). This concentration corresponds to a pH of 7.40 (by definition pH $= -\log_{10} [H^+]$). The pH of some specialized fluids in the body can be very different from that of blood. For example, the pH of the acidic gastric juice is about 1 ($[H^+] = 10^8$ nEq $\cdot$ l^{-1}), and that of the somewhat alkaline pancreatic fluid is about 8 ($[H^+] = 10$ nEq $\cdot$ l^{-1}). The pH scale is convenient to use when discussing $[H^+]$ because wide-ranging $[H^+]$ values are easily expressed by the compressed pH scale. In the context of the pH scale it is interesting that pH electrodes employed to measure $[H^+]$ do so by developing an electrical potential that is directly proportional to the logarithm of the $[H^+]$. It is important to keep in mind that when $[H^+]$ goes up, pH goes down, and vice versa, and that the two scales are not linearly related to one another.

H^+ concentration in blood is less than a millionth that of Na^+ (Na^+ is about 140 milliEq $\cdot$ l^{-1} or mEq $\cdot$ l^{-1}). Why be so concerned about a substance that is in such low concentration in arterial blood? The reason is that deviations in $[H^+]$ from normal can have deleterious effects on a variety of systems. The heart is compromised by acidosis; it depresses myocardial activity and interferes with agents that normally stimulate the heart. Moreover, defibrillation is harder to accomplish in acidosis, and cardiac arrhythmias occur more often. Elevated $[H^+]$ within the brain is very harmful to central nervous system function, impairing mental abilities and ultimately causing coma and death. Within the body enzymatic systems are also sensitive to $[H^+]$. Thus, if $[H^+]$ becomes too high (acidosis) or too low (alkalosis), death can result. The range of $[H^+]$ values compatible with life is approximately 16 nEq $\cdot$ l^{-1} (pH = 7.8) to 100 nEq $\cdot$ l^{-1} (pH = 7.0).

Regulation of H^+ involves two physiological systems. The rapidly acting system in acid–base homeostasis is the pulmonary system. In fact, the result of gaseous CO_2 elimination or retention by the lungs upon H^+ regulation is such that CO_2 can be considered as a volatile (gaseous) acid. The slowly acting system is the renal system. In the latter, H^+ is eliminated or retained through alterations in bicarbonate reabsorption by the kidneys. In this way, the kidneys affect acid–base homeostasis by altering the excretion of nonvolatile acids.

Useful Definitions

To understand acid–base regulation, it is important first to know the meanings of certain terms.

1. An *acid* is defined as a proton donor. HCl, for instance, is a strong acid because it dissociates readily into H^+ and Cl^- when it is dissolved in water:

$$HCl \rightarrow H^+ + Cl^-$$

2. A *base* is defined as a proton acceptor. NaOH is an example of a strong base because it readily and completely dissociates into OH^- (the proton acceptor) and Na^+:

$$NaOH \rightarrow Na^+ + OH^-$$

3. A *weak acid* or *weak base* is an acid or base that incompletely dissociates. Carbonic acid, for instance, undergoes the following reversible equilibrium reaction:

$$H_2CO_3 \underset{}{\overset{K_{H_2CO_3}}{\rightleftharpoons}} H^+ + HCO_3^-$$

$K_{H_2CO_3}$ is the dissociation constant and relates at equilibrium the concentrations of the three species in the following reaction:

$$K_{H_2CO_3} = \frac{[H^+][HCO_3^-]}{[H_2CO_3]} \tag{13.1}$$

NOTE:

$$pK_{H_2CO_3} = -\log_{10}(K_{H_2CO_3}) = pH -\log_{10}\frac{[HCO_3^-]}{[H_2CO_3]} \qquad (13.2)$$

4. A *buffer* reduces the changes in pH resulting from the addition of strong acids or bases to a solution. For example, a buffer system consisting of a weak acid, HA (HA is simply used here to designate the general weak acid) and its salt, A⁻, can be described by the following equilibrium reaction:

$$HA \rightleftharpoons H^+ + A^-$$

From this reaction it is apparent that if more and more H⁺ is added to the system, then some of it will combine with A⁻ to form HA. Thus the amount of H⁺ present at equilibrium will be less than when A⁻ is absent from the solution. Another important feature is that a buffer does its best buffering over a range of [H⁺] where the concentrations of HA and A⁻ are of the same order of magnitude. This can be very significant when one considers which of the many buffer systems in the body will contribute significantly to *in vivo* buffering. Thus for buffer systems to be effective in plasma they must have characteristic dissociations such that weak acids or bases and their corresponding salts are each of comparable concentrations at the normal plasma pH of approximately 7.4.

Buffering

As stated, buffering reduces the changes in [H⁺] that occur with the addition of strong acids or bases to a solution. To illustrate this concept, consider the effects of the presence or absence of 100 mmoles of NaAc on the concentration of H⁺ following the addition of 1 mmole of HCl to 1 liter of water. The following set of reactions takes place:

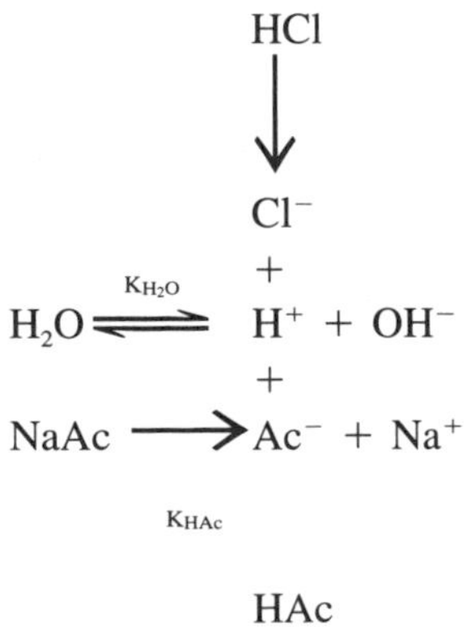

$$HCl$$
$$\downarrow$$
$$Cl^-$$
$$+$$
$$H_2O \underset{K_{H_2O}}{\rightleftharpoons} H^+ + OH^-$$
$$+$$
$$NaAc \longrightarrow Ac^- + Na^+$$
$$\scriptsize K_{HAc}$$
$$HAc$$

Utilization of the various equilibrium dissociation relationships and the electrical neutrality relationship results in an equation (not illustrated) that describes $[H^+]$ as a function of the initial NaAc concentration (this is the value of $[Na^+]$) and the HCl concentration (this is the value of $[Cl^-]$). If this equation is solved for the case where 100 mmoles of NaAc and 1 mmmole of HCl are dissolved in 1 liter of H_2O, the result is an $[H^+]$ of 1.78×10^{-7} Eq $\cdot$ l^{-1} or a pH of 6.75. In the absence of the buffer the pH for this amount of HCl is 3. Thus the presence of NaAc greatly reduces the amount of free H^+ in solution.

Next, consider the example cited where 100 mmoles of NaAc is added to 1 liter of H_2O, but now start at a pH of 4.75 where one-half of the acetate ion in NaAc is in the form of free Ac^- and the other half is undissociated as HAc (this point was chosen because at this condition pH = pK_{HAc}; see Eq. 13.2). Figure 13.1 shows the effect of adding additional HCl and also NaOH to this solution. The resulting S-shaped curve shown in Figure 13.1 is the titration curve for this buffer system. The slope (dashed line in Fig. 13.1) that measures the change in pH for each mEq of strong acid or base added is smallest for pH values near the pK; thus the best buffering will occur here.

Another useful concept that is helpful in assessing buffering capability is that of the buffer value. The buffer value is the negative of the reciprocal of the slope of the titration curve. Therefore, buffer value has dimensions of mEq $\cdot$ pH unit^{-1}, and this is simply referred to as the *slyke* (sl), in honor of D. D. Van Slyke, who was a pioneer researcher in this field. It is evident that buffer value is the amount of H^+ (expressed in mEq) that can be added or removed from a solution for each

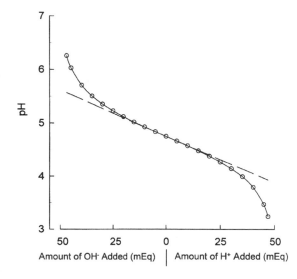

Figure 13.1. Titration curve for an NaAc buffer system. The buffer consisted of 100 mmoles of NaAc dissolved in 1 liter of H_2O. The titration curve is the **solid line** joining the open circles. The slope at the point of best buffering (pH = pK_{HAc}), the highest buffer value, is indicated by the **dashed line.**

unit change in pH. Thus the shallower the slope of the titration curve, the higher will be the buffer value, and therefore the greater the buffering capacity of a buffer system. For the system illustrated in Figure 13.1, the maximum buffer value is 57.5 sl at a pH of 4.75.

Buffering in the Body

Now that we have developed some basic concepts regarding acid–base chemistry, we can apply these to consider buffering within the body. The body contains in its various compartments a number of buffer systems. Table 13.1 summarizes the important systems. The two most important buffers are $H_2PO_4^-$ and the imidazole ring of the amino acid histidine because their pK values are close to the physiological range of pH. Thus proteins that contain histidine will function as good buffers; this includes the histidine residues that are present on the hemoglobin molecule.

For each buffer system the following relationship can be written, based on the general dissociation equilibrium for a buffer:

$$pH = pK + \log_{10} \frac{[H^+ \text{ acceptor}]}{[\text{weak acid}]} \tag{13.3}$$

The $[H^+]$ can be determined from the ratio of the concentrations of the basic form (H^+ acceptor) to the weak acidic form of each buffer. Clearly, all of the body's buffer systems shown in Table 13.1 are not independent of one another, but are

Table 13.1. Important Buffer Systems of the Body

COMPARTMENT	WEAK ACID FORM/H+ ACCEPTOR
Plasma and extracellular fluid	H_2CO_3/HCO_3^- $H_2PO_4^-/HPO_4^=$
Red blood cells	HHb/Hb$^-$
Intracellular fluid	$H_2PO_4^-/HPO_4^=$ HPr/Pr$^-$
Bone	$HCO_3^-/CO_3^=$ $H_2PO_4^-/HPO_4^=$

Hb designates the hemoglobin molecule; Pr designates protein, and buffering is associated with the imidazole ring of the amino acid histidine.

linked at least in part through [H$^+$]. This concept of interdependence is referred to as the *isohydric principle*. It also means that changes in the ratio of base to weak acid forms of any one of the buffers will determine the [H$^+$] and thereby also the ratio of the two forms of all other buffers in solution. This has important implications for the study of acids and bases in the body. It means that we can look at any one of the buffer systems and use this as a window into the pH of the various fluid compartments of body. In clinical practice it is convenient to use the bicarbonate system as such a window because measurements in this system can readily be made.

Bicarbonate System

To understand the bicarbonate system, consider the following dissociation that occurs between its weak acid, carbonic acid (H$_2$CO$_3$), and its conjugate base, HCO$_3^-$:

$$H_2CO_3 \xrightleftharpoons{K_{H_2CO_3}} H^+ + HCO_3^-$$

$$K_{H_2CO_3} = \frac{[H^+][HCO_3^-]}{[H_2CO_3]} \tag{13.4}$$

Solving for [H$^+$] yields

$$[H^+] = K_{H_2CO_3} \frac{[H_2CO_3]}{[HCO_3^-]} \tag{13.5}$$

Taking the logarithm of both sides of this relationship and converting [H$^+$] to pH (as in Eq. 13.3) results in

$$pH = pK_{H_2CO_3} + \log \frac{[HCO_3^-]}{[H_2CO_3]} \tag{13.6}$$

This is the well-known *Henderson-Hasselbalch equation*. What it makes clear is that the ratio of [HCO$_3^-$] to [H$_2$CO$_3$] determines the pH. If [HCO$_3^-$] increases, for example, then the pH will rise and the solution will become more alkaline; if [HCO$_3^-$] falls, the solution will become more acid.

The buffering ability of the bicarbonate system, like that of other buffer systems, can be assessed by adding H$^+$ and determining its buffer value. For this system changes in [HCO$_3^-$] will equal the amount of [H$^+$] added to or removed from the solution. Alternatively, in terms of buffer value, we can write

$$\text{Buffer value} = -\frac{\Delta[HCO_3^-]}{\Delta pH} \tag{13.7}$$

In the presence of the enzyme carbonic anhydrase (CA), CO_2 can be readily hydrated to H_2CO_3. As a result, the bicarbonate buffer system is more completely described by the following two sets of equilibria:

$$CO_2 + H_2O \overset{CA}{\rightleftharpoons} H_2CO_3 \rightleftharpoons H^+ + HCO_3^-$$

By combining these two equilibria and assuming that the concentration of H_2O is constant at 55.5 moles $\cdot$ l^{-1}, we can derive the following Henderson-Hasselbalch type of relationship for this system:

$$pH = pK + \log \frac{[HCO_3^-]}{[CO_2]} \tag{13.8}$$

At body temperature the pK for this expression is 6.1. Even though the pK is 1.3 units less than that of the normal blood pH, the bicarbonate system can still function as a good physiological buffer. Because P_{CO_2} is customarily measured with a P_{CO_2} electrode, rather than the total CO_2 concentration, the P_{CO_2} must be multiplied by its solubility to determine the $[CO_2]$ in the above relationship. Use of the solubility value shown in Eq. 6.6 ($\beta CO_2 = 0.072$ ml $\cdot$ dl^{-1} $\cdot$ mm Hg^{-1}) and conversion of this to the appropriate concentration units yields

$$pH = 6.1 + \log \frac{[HCO_3^-]}{[0.03\ P_{CO_2}]} \tag{13.9}$$

In this relationship $[HCO_3^-]$ is expressed in units of mEq $\cdot$ l^{-1} and P_{CO_2} in mm Hg.

Equation 13.9 can be used to calculate the pH of arterial blood. In normal arterial blood $[HCO_3^-]$ is 24 mEq $\cdot$ l^{-1} and the P_{CO_2} is 40 mm Hg. These values yield the normal arterial pH of 7.40. From this Henderson-Hasselbalch relationship it is apparent that if one knows the value of any two of the variables ($[H^+]$, $[HCO_3^-]$, or P_{CO_2}), the third can be calculated.

This relationship, depicted in a *Davenport diagram*, is shown in Figure 13.2. Here the y-axis is the $[HCO_3^-]$ and the x-axis is the pH. The curved lines in Figure 13.2 are for different, but constant, P_{CO_2} values. Because P_{CO_2} is a constant for each line, these are called *isobars*, meaning lines of constant pressure. Thus each point on the various isobars shown in Figure 13.2 is a unique solution to the above

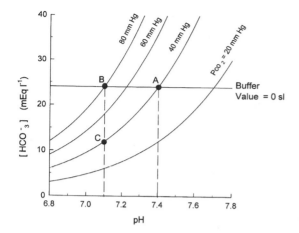

Figure 13.2. Davenport diagram showing the relationship between [HCO$_3^-$], pH, and P$_{CO_2}$. The lines were derived by the solution of the Henderson-Hasselbalch relationship for the bicarbonate system. Also shown is the line corresponding to a buffer value of 0 sl. For a pure bicarbonate buffer system, starting at point A and raising P$_{CO_2}$ from 40 to 80 mm Hg results in little production of HCO$_3^-$ but a drop in pH from 7.4 to 7.1 (point B). Point C indicates the HCO$_3^-$ and pH values when H$^+$ is added to the system while maintaining a P$_{CO_2}$ of 40 mm Hg.

Henderson-Hasselbalch type of relationship. An alternative graphical representation of this system that is also used in clinical practise is the *Siggaard-Andersen nomogram*. In this case, the y-axis is the P$_{CO_2}$, the x-axis is the pH, and lines of constant [HCO$_3^-$] are plotted within the P$_{CO_2}$–pH plane. Both representations contain the same information, and it is a matter of preference which one is used. In this book we use the Davenport diagram.

What happens if the only buffer system present is the bicarbonate system and the P$_{CO_2}$ is increased from its initial value of 40 mm Hg so that the pH drops from 7.4 to 7.1? In this case the change in [H$^+$] is 39 nEq · l^{-1}. For each H$^+$ added, a HCO$_3^-$ is formed so the change in [HCO$_3^-$] also will be 39 nEq · l^{-1}. The [HCO$_3^-$] will rise imperceptibly from its initial value of 24.000000 mEq · l^{-1} to 24.000039 mEq · l^{-1}. Thus changes in P$_{CO_2}$ do not materially change the [HCO$_3^-$] for this system*. The buffer value can be calculated:

$$\text{Buffer value} = -\frac{\Delta[\text{HCO}_3^-]}{\Delta\text{pH}} = -\frac{39 \times 10^{-6}\ \text{mEq} \cdot \text{l}^{-1}}{-0.3\ \text{pH units}} \cong 0\ \text{sl} \qquad (13.10)$$

*Actually [HCO$_3^-$] will rise by 329 nEq · l^{-1} because OH$^-$ in H$_2$O will buffer the H$^+$ formed. This additional buffering does not change the conclusion that changes in P$_{CO_2}$ do not materially change the [HCO$_3^-$] in the system because the starting [HCO$_3^-$] is so high compared with the change in [HCO$_3^-$] that occurs.

From such a small buffer value it can be concluded that the bicarbonate buffer system *alone* is a poor buffer for hydrogen ion increases arising from P_{CO_2} increases.

To determine the exact value of P_{CO_2} when the pH is 7.1, we again use the Henderson-Hasselbalch relationship, which yields a P_{CO_2} value of 80 mm Hg. Thus, raising the P_{CO_2} from 40 to 80 mm Hg causes the pH to fall from 7.4 to 7.1 (a 39 nEq $\cdot$ l^{-1} rise in $[H^+]$). Figure 13.2 also illustrates this relationship on the Davenport diagram. The point marked A is the starting point, and the horizontal line through A describes the $[HCO_3^-]$–pH of the pure bicarbonate system for increases and decreases in P_{CO_2} from its starting value of 40 mm Hg. The point labeled B is where the P_{CO_2} is 80 mm Hg and the pH is 7.1. The horizontal line through points A and B is the titration line for this system with a zero slope or a buffer value of 0 sl.

Now consider what happens to the bicarbonate buffer system if H^+ is added to or subtracted from the system by addition of a strong acid or base and P_{CO_2} held fixed at 40 mm Hg. In this isocapnic situation the final pH of the system will be described by points along the P_{CO_2} = 40 mm Hg isobar. Figure 13.2 illustrates this example where a fixed acid is added and the pH drops to 7.1 (point C), resulting in a substantial drop in $[HCO_3^-]$ from its initial value of 24 to 12 mEq $\cdot$ l^{-1}. Movement of the acid–base status along the P_{CO_2} = 40 mm Hg isobar is indicative of acid–base states of either metabolic acidosis (movement downward and to the left) or metabolic alkalosis (movement upward and to the right). The term *metabolic* refers to acids and bases that are noncarbonic in origin. Among such metabolic acids are lactic, phosphoric, and sulfuric acids.

Bicarbonate System *In Vivo*

When P_{CO_2} is increased or decreased within the body, changes in $[HCO_3^-]$ are not equal to changes in $[H^+]$ because other buffer systems are present besides the bicarbonate system, such as the hemoglobin buffer system. The following equilibria describe these two interacting buffer systems:

$$CO_2 + H_2O \overset{CA}{\rightleftharpoons} H_2CO_3 \rightleftharpoons H^+ + HCO_3^-$$

$$+$$

$$Hb^-$$

$$HHb$$

From this it is evident that as more and more CO_2 is added, more H^+ and

HCO_3^- will be produced. In turn, the H^+ produced will be buffered by the Hb^-. Thus at equilibrium, the change in $[HCO_3^-]$ will be much greater than the change in $[H^+]$.

Hemoglobin is an effective buffer because (*1*) it is in high concentration in red blood cells; (*2*) because imidazole groups are present on the hemoglobin molecule, the pK of hemoglobin (6.8) is close to the normal blood pH range; and (*3*) hemoglobin O_2 saturation alters the buffering capacity of hemoglobin. Where P_{O_2} is low, as in the systemic capillaries, the H^+ affinity is high; the converse occurs in the pulmonary capillaries where the P_{O_2} is high.

Before considering *in vivo* buffering by the bicarbonate system, we need it to understand the effect of hemoglobin on the buffering by HCO_3^- when this is assessed in a beaker of blood. This beaker will contain both hemoglobin and HCO_3^- buffer systems. If we begin by bubbling the beaker with air containing a P_{CO_2} of 40 mm Hg, the pH will be 7.4 and the $[HCO_3^-]$, 24 mEq $\cdot$ l^{-1}. If the P_{CO_2} is then raised to 80 mm Hg by increasing its partial pressure in the air being bubbled, at equilibrium the pH will be 7.20 (an $[H^+]$ of 63 nEq $\cdot$ l^{-1}) and the $[HCO_3^-]$, 30 mEq $\cdot$ l^{-1}. It is evident that hemoglobin has dramatically increased the buffering capacity of this bicarbonate system. Recall that without hemoglobin, the pH dropped to 7.10 (an $[H^+]$ of 79 nEq $\cdot$ l^{-1}); thus hemoglobin has reduced the increase in $[H^+]$ by 41%. The better buffering ability of blood can be quantitatively expressed in terms of the buffer value:

$$\text{Buffer value} = -\frac{\Delta[HCO_3^-]}{\Delta pH} = \frac{(30 - 24)\ mEq \cdot l^{-1}}{(7.2 - 7.4)\ pH\ units} = 30\ sl \quad (13.11)$$

Figure 13.3 illustrates the differences in the buffering abilities of these two systems: the bicarbonate system alone where buffer value = 0 sl and the bicarbonate and hemoglobin systems together where the buffer value = 30 sl. Starting from point A and elevating P_{CO_2} to 80 mm Hg, Figure 13.3 shows that, for blood, point C will be reached. The line joining points A and C has a slope of 30 sl—this high value indicates an elevated buffering ability of blood. The slope of this line depends on the hemoglobin concentration in the blood. At 30 sl it represents a normal hemoglobin concentration of 15 gms $\cdot$ dl of blood^{-1}. If the hemoglobin concentration rises, as in the case of polycythemia, the slope will steepen; conversely, if the concentration falls, as in the case of anemia, the slope will decline. The consequences of such alterations on the buffering ability of blood are easily appreciated by considering Figure 13.3.

This example of acid–base behavior of blood studied in isolation as it responds to alterations in P_{CO_2} is obviously an artifactual one. In the body there are interacting fluid compartments, only one of which is blood. The consequences of this are

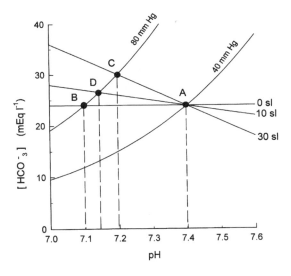

Figure 13.3. Davenport diagram showing the effects of different buffer values on the resulting pH when P_{CO_2} is raised from 40 to 80 mm Hg. The higher the buffer value, the better the buffering, as shown by the smaller change in pH from its initial value of 7.4.

related to the volume of the compartments as well as the buffers contained within each one. Blood makes up about one-third of the extracellular fluid volume; the remaining two-thirds is the interstitial fluid volume. The acid–base behavior of the interstitial fluid, which has a buffer value of 0 sl, is like that of a pure bicarbonate solution. Thus the overall acid–base response of the extracellular fluid (ecf) can be determined by considering the relative volumes of both components:

$$\text{Buffer value}_{ecf} = \tfrac{1}{3} \times 30 \text{ sl} + \tfrac{2}{3} \times 0 \text{ sl} = 10 \text{ sl} \qquad (13.12)$$

Figure 13.3 illustrates the effect of reducing the buffer value to 10 sl on the buffering ability of blood. It shows that the final pH (point D) will be 7.14 (72 nEq · l⁻¹) when the P_{CO_2} is raised from 40 to 80 mm Hg and that [HCO₃⁻] will rise from 24 to 26.5 mEq · l⁻¹. The line of slope of 10 sl is very important because it describes the steady-state acid–base status when changes are made in P_{CO_2}. Points along this line with increasing P_{CO_2}, from a normal starting value of 40 mm Hg, describe conditions of respiratory acidosis like those that result from hypoventilation. Points along the 10 sl line with decreasing P_{CO_2} describe conditions of respiratory alkalosis such as those that result from hyperventilation. From the projection of this line onto the y-axis, one can predict the extent of changes in [HCO₃⁻] stemming from uncompensated respiratory alterations that may arise in different respiratory diseases. Thus during conditions of respiratory acid–base disturbances, the arterial [HCO₃⁻] will be somewhere in the range of 21 to 27 mEq · l⁻¹.

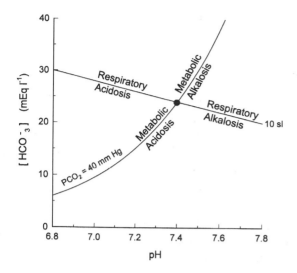

Figure 13.4. Davenport diagram showing the consequences of uncompensated respiratory and metabolic acid–base disturbances.

Figure 13.4 summarizes the different conditions of uncompensated respiratory acidosis and alkalosis, as well as uncompensated metabolic acidosis and alkalosis.

Base Excess

The concept of *base excess* (BE) provides a useful tool for assessing the magnitude of metabolic acid–base abnormalities in the presence of *in vivo* buffering. The greater the deviation of the BE from its normal range of ± 3 mEq $\cdot$ l^{-1}, in either the positive direction with metabolic alkalosis or the negative direction with metabolic acidosis, the greater is the extent of the acid–base abnormality. These ideas can be summarized as follows:

Metabolic alkalosis: BE > 3 mEq $\cdot$ l^{-1}
No underlying metabolic acid–base abnormality: BE $= \pm 3$ mEq $\cdot$ l^{-1}
Metabolic acidosis: BE < -3 mEq $\cdot$ l^{-1}

In calculating the BE, one adds or subtracts CO_2 to return the pH of arterial blood to normal (7.40). Base excess in mEq $\cdot$ l^{-1} is the difference of the new [HCO$_3^-$] at the pH of 7.4 from the normal [HCO$_3^-$] of 24 mEq $\cdot$ l^{-1}, and it indicates the type and extent of metabolic acid–base abnormality. Effectively, the procedure for calculating the BE is a titration that uses addition or subtraction of CO_2 as a respiratory acid or base to correct the pH to normal. We have already seen that *in vivo* this titration can be described on the Davenport diagram along a line whose slope is -10 sl.

Pure Metabolic Acidosis

To understand the concept of BE, consider the example in Figure 13.5 where the arterial pH = 7.20, $[HCO_3^-]$ = 15.1 mEq $\cdot$ l^{-1}, and the P_{CO_2} = 40 mm Hg. Point A indicates the normal arterial blood acid–base status, and point B is the acid–base status in this example. To return the subject's pH to normal (thereby reducing $[H^+]$) requires a *conceptual* hyperventilation. This is easy to remember by recalling the bicarbonate system equilibria shown earlier. Starting at point B, the subject's P_{CO_2} will be reduced along a line whose slope is $-$ 10 sl. C is the final point in this procedure because it is here that the pH has returned to its normal value of 7.40. To calculate the $[HCO_3^-]$ at this point, all we need to know is that the slope of the line connecting point B and C is $-$ 10 sl. Thus:

$$\text{Buffer value} = -\frac{\Delta[HCO_3^-]}{\Delta pH} = 10 \text{ sl}$$

$$\Delta[HCO_3^-] = -10 \times \Delta pH = -10(7.4 - 7.2) = -2 \text{ mEq} \cdot l^{-1}$$

At point C $[HCO_3^-]$ = 15.1 $-$ 2 = 13.1 mEq $\cdot$ l^{-1}

BE = 13.1 $-$ 24 $\cong$ -11 mEq $\cdot$ l^{-1}

From this we can conclude that the initial arterial blood conditions are those

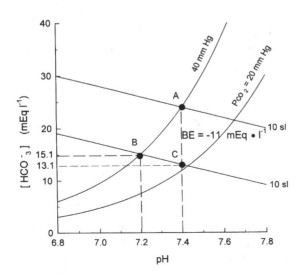

Figure 13.5. Davenport diagram showing the procedure for determining the base excess (BE) for the case of uncompensated metabolic acidosis (point B). See text for discussion.

of a person with metabolic acidosis because the BE is less than -3 mEq $\cdot$ l^{-1} . Among the diseases that cause metabolic acidosis are severe diarrhea, (where there is a loss of bicarbonate from the bowel,) diabetic ketoacidosis, and kidney diseases (where the H^+ secretion mechanism fails).

A question that often arises when the concept of BE is applied to determine the acid-base status of a subject is, how do you know the sign of the change in $[HCO_3^-]$ without keeping track of the sign in the calculations shown above? An easy way to remember whether $[HCO_3^-]$ will go up or down when the pH is corrected to 7.4 is to recall the following equilibrium reactions:

$$CO_2 + H_2O \overset{CA}{\rightleftharpoons} H_2CO_3 \rightleftharpoons H^+ + HCO_3^-$$

If CO_2 is reduced so as to reduce the $[H^+]$, the $[HCO_3^-]$ will decrease; conversely, if we increase CO_2 to raise the $[H^+]$, the $[HCO_3^-]$ will increase. Thus the sign of the change in $[HCO_3^-]$ can easily be determined.

Determining the BE also permits clinicians to calculate the dose of administered base that is required to correct a patient's base deficit. This correction is empirical but nonetheless useful. It is equal to the BE multiplied by 30% of the body weight in kg. In the example of metabolic acidosis given above, the amount of base, such as $[HCO_3^-]$, that needs to be administered to a 70 kg subject is

$$HCO_3^- = 11 \times 0.3 \times 70 = 230 \text{ mEq of } HCO_3^-$$

This amount of HCO_3^- does not take into account acid–base changes of the intracellular compartment. Because it is just a therapeutic estimate, frequent measurements of the arterial blood acid–base status should be made to determine the correctness of any dose.

Pure Respiratory Acidosis

Another example will serve to illustrate the utility of BE. Consider a person with pure respiratory acidosis in whom the P_{CO_2} has risen to 60 mm Hg due to hypoventilation and the pH has fallen to 7.25. The $[HCO_3^-]$ will be 25.5 mEq $\cdot$ l^{-1}. Figure 13.6 illustrates this condition by means of a Davenport diagram. Point B is the initial acid-base status of the subject. To calculate the BE, the pH must first be raised ($[H^+]$ decreased) by conceptually hyperventilating the subject to lower the P_{CO_2}, and this will drive the pH to 7.4. As before, the subject's acid–base status during this conceptual procedure will be described along a line whose slope is -10 sl. Point A is the final point in this procedure because at this point the pH

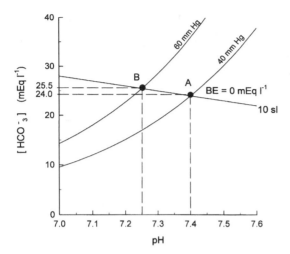

Figure 13.6. Davenport diagram showing the procedure for determining the base excess ([BE] which is zero in this instance) for the case of uncompensated respiratory acidosis (point B). See text for discussion.

is 7.40. Obviously, we need to go no further because at this point the $[HCO_3^-]$ is 24 mEq $\cdot$ l^{-1} and therefore the BE is 0. We can prove this rigorously by the following:

$$\text{Buffer value} = -\frac{\Delta[HCO_3^-]}{\Delta pH} = 10 \text{ sl}$$

$$\Delta[HCO_3^-] = -10 \times \Delta pH = -10(7.4 - 7.25) = -1.5 \text{ mEq} \cdot l^{-1}$$

At point A $[HCO_3^-] = 25.5 - 1.5 = 24.0$ mEq $\cdot$ l^{-1}

BE $= 24.0 - 24.0 = 0$ mEq $\cdot$ l^{-1}

Because the BE indicates the magnitude of the metabolic and not the respiratory acid–base abnormality, a BE of 0 indicates that there was not an underlying metabolic acid–base problem, but simply a respiratory acidosis.

Combined Disorders and Compensation Mechanisms

Respiratory and metabolic acid–base abnormalities sometimes coexist. For example, during asphyxia there is acute respiratory acidosis due to a reduction in alveolar ventilation, and this may coexist with acute metabolic acidosis due to hypoxia-induced lactic acidosis.

Combined states of acid–base abnormality can also occur when a primary acid–base abnormality activates a compensatory mechanism designed to alleviate the initial acid–base derangement. The function of the compensation is to return the arterial pH toward normal. Clinically this is seen, for example, in diabetic ketoacidosis where the initial metabolic acidosis causes a ventilatory compensation; this is described next.

Ventilatory Compensation

Through its effect on $P_{A_{CO_2}}$ the ventilatory control system (see Chapter 9) compensates for a primary metabolic acid–base disturbance. For example, in response to primary metabolic acidosis, there is a compensatory ventilatory hyperventilation that reduces arterial P_{CO_2}, thereby reducing the degree of acidosis. Metabolic alkalosis produces hypoventilation. This will cause the arterial P_{CO_2} to rise, thereby reducing the degree of alkalosis. Ventilatory compensations for primary metabolic acid–base disturbances occur rapidly, usually over the course of minutes to hours. Unfortunately, they are usually not complete, that is, they do not return the arterial pH all the way to 7.40. The mechanism of these compensations relies on the stimulation of chemoreceptors by the increase in arterial [H$^+$] (see Chapter 9 for a discussion of the basis for this ventilatory stimulation). Figure 13.7 shows the extent

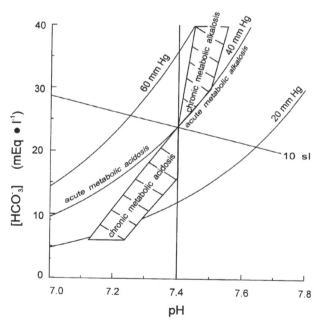

Figure 13.7. Davenport diagram showing the response to both acute and chronic (compensated) metabolic acidosis and alkalosis. The closed areas with diagonal lines are the zones showing the chronic acid–base values.

of both the acute and chronic (following ventilatory compensation) responses to metabolic acidosis and alkalosis.

Renal Compensation

In response to a primary respiratory acid–base disturbance, the kidney retains or excretes [HCO_3^-] and this affects arterial pH. This permits almost complete compensation of the primary respiratory acid base disturbance. Renal compensation takes place over a long period of time, usually days. In severe respiratory acidosis, when the Pa_{CO_2} is higher than about 70 mm Hg, the compensation does not return the arterial pH to near 7.4. In this case, the [HCO_3^-] reabsorption by the kidneys reaches a maximum, and this restricts the degree of compensation. For the excretion of H^+ in urine, as during compensation for respiratory acidosis, the H^+ in the kidney tubular fluid combines with NH_3 to form NH_4^+ and with $HPO_4^=$ to form $H_2PO_4^-$. These ions act as buffers for H^+ in urine and increase its effective excretion. In primary respiratory alkalosis (e.g., due to chronic hyperventilation) there is increased secretion of HCO_3^- by the kidneys. Figure 13.8 shows both the acute

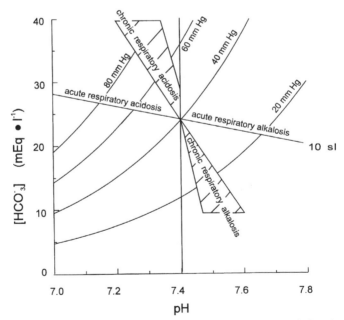

Figure 13.8. Davenport diagram showing the response to both acute and chronic (compensated) respiratory acidosis and alkalosis. The closed areas with diagonal lines are the zones showing the chronic acid–base values.

and chronic (following renal compensation) responses to respiratory acidosis and alkalosis.

Another way of understanding these compensations is to recall that it is the ratio of $[HCO_3^-]:P_{CO_2}$ that determines the pHa. Thus, in respiratory derangements, it is the P_{CO_2} that is initially altered, and it follows that subsequently $[HCO_3^-]$ would need to be changed in the same direction by the compensation to return the pHa to normal. Similarly, in metabolic derangements the $[HCO_3^-]$ is initially changed, and subsequently the P_{CO_2} would need to be changed in the same direction by the compensation to restore the pHa to normal.

Further Reading

1. Davenport HW. *The ABC of Acid–Base Chemistry*, 6th ed. Chicago: The University of Chicago Press, 1974.
2. Effros RM, Windell JL. Acid–base balance. In: Murray JF, Nadel JA, editors. *Textbook of Respiratory Medicine*, 2nd ed. Philadelphia: WB Saunders, 1994, pp175–198.
3. Goldfarb S, Sharma K. Acid–base balance. In: Fishman AP, editor. *Pulmonary Diseases and Disorders,* 3rd ed. New York: McGraw Hill, 1998, pp 207–220.
4. Woodbury JW. Body acid-base state and its regulation. In: Patton HD, Fuchs AF, Hille B, Scher AM, Steiner R, editors. *Textbook of Physiology,* 21st ed, vol 2. Philadelphia: WB Saunders, 1989, pp 1114–1138.

Study Questions

13.1. What is a buffer value?

13.2. Name four important buffer systems in the body.

13.3. Why is hemoglobin an effective buffer?

13.4. When P_{CO_2} is changed, why will a larger change in pH occur for blood *in vivo* than for blood *in vitro*?

13.5. In response to chronic respiratory acidosis a metabolic compensation normally occurs. How does plasma bicarbonate change during this compensation?

13.6. Ventilatory compensation in response to chronic metabolic acidosis is not of itself capable of fully returning the pH of arterial blood to 7.4. Why is this compensation not complete?

13.7. If a patient's arterial blood has a P_{CO_2} of 30 mm Hg and an $[HCO_3^-]$ of 15 mEq· l^{-1}, what is the patient's base excess?

14

Comparative Respiratory Physiology

The study of comparative respiratory physiology provides a broad and useful perspective on the respiratory physiology of humans. One of the first observations is that the function of the respiratory system can be accomplished in several different ways. Each way of functioning appears to be ideally suited to the environment and behavior of the species in question. Each particular respiratory system has evolved to provide optimal efficiency for gas exchange under the behavioral and environmental conditions of an organism.

The essential purpose of the respiratory system in any species is the exchange of O_2 and CO_2. As we have seen, the respiratory system has other functions, but these are not dealt with in this chapter. In very small organisms, the exchange of gas can be carried out by simple diffusion. When the surface area-to-volume ratio is large and the diffusion distances are small, diffusion is all that is needed. As diffusion distances get longer, however, convective mechanisms must be used. Notable exceptions to this rule are the insects. Air is conducted into the body through spiracles, or long narrow tubes, that pass from the exoskeleton into and throughout the body. These are sufficient to exchange gas even in these insects that have high metabolic demands due to prolonged or rapid flight.

Larger species use a combination of convection and diffusion to exchange O_2 and CO_2. The outside breathing medium (either air or water) is brought into or through the respiratory apparatus by convection. Gases exchange with blood via diffusion through the barrier separating the air or water from blood. Blood transports gas between the respiratory apparatus and the respiring tissues. Figure 14.1 illustrates the roles of convection and diffusion in several types of gas-exchanging organs. Each type of respiratory organ accomplishes the task in a different way that is suited to the animal's behavior and gas exchange requirements.

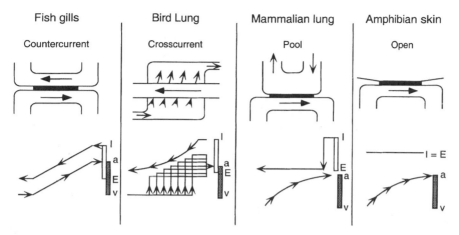

Figure 14.1 Different gas exchange system configurations. The countercurrent system of the fish gill allows arterial blood leaving the gill to have a P_{O_2} greater than the water leaving the gill. The cross-current system of the bird lung also provides a means for arterial blood P_{O_2} to exceed exhaled gas P_{O_2} by a small amount. The pool system of the mammalian lung provides for efficient gas exchange with an arterial P_{O_2} that is close to, but does not exceed, alveolar P_{O_2}. The open system of the amphibian skin is inefficient because of diffusion limitation, with arterial P_{O_2} being lower than outside air P_{O_2}. The lower figures represent inspired (I), expired (E), arterial (a), and venous (v) P_{O_2} values. (Adapted from Piiper J, Scheid P. Comparative physiology of respiration: Functional analysis of gas exchange organs in vertebrates. In: Widdecombe JG, editor. *International Review of Physiology: Respiratory Physiology II*, vol 14. Boston: University Park Press, 1977, pp 220–253.)

Gills

Water breathing presents significant challenges for the fish. Physical properties of water present four major gas exchange problems: (*1*) higher viscosity of water resulting in higher frictional energy loss during locomotion; (*2*) higher density of water resulting in an increased energy cost of acceleration; (*3*) lower diffusivity of O_2 in water versus air; and (*4*) low solubility of O_2 in water compared with air. Gills are well adapted for gas exchange in a water environment. They allow fish to expose blood to the external medium. The convective flow of water provides O_2 and takes away CO_2. The availability of large quantities of water also allows the gills to carry out osmotic regulation, exchanging ions and water with the external environment.

Gas exchange by gills is limited in the external medium by the lower diffusivity of gases in water compared with air. Gill anatomy, however, allows the fish to overcome diffusion problems. The gill surface area is large and is arranged as a series of lamella on a series of arches (Fig. 14.2). This large surface area increases the diffusing capacity of both O_2 and CO_2 (Fick's law, Chapter 1).

Blood flows through the gill lamella in the opposite direction of water flow, setting up a countercurrent gas exchange process. This allows a greater exchange of gas than would be possible in a cocurrent system, where blood and water flow in the same direction. Figure 14.3 is a schematic representation of P_{O_2} in both water and blood in the gill lamella. Blood entering the lamella encounters water with a high P_{O_2}—not as high as the incoming water, but high enough to provide O_2. The driving force for O_2 exchange at any point in the lamella is the difference in P_{O_2} between water and blood at that point. As blood progresses through the capillary, it comes in contact with water containing still higher P_{O_2}, allowing further uptake of O_2. Along the entire length of the capillary, blood continues to take up O_2, eventually reaching P_{O_2} values that are close to the incoming P_{O_2} of the water. This system provides for a very high extraction of O_2 from the water and a high arterial P_{O_2}. Contrast this with a cocurrent system where the effluent blood could not achieve a P_{O_2} higher than that of the effluent water, thus reducing the extraction of O_2 from water and the P_{O_2} in blood.

Mammals are unable to survive breathing water for several reasons: The high

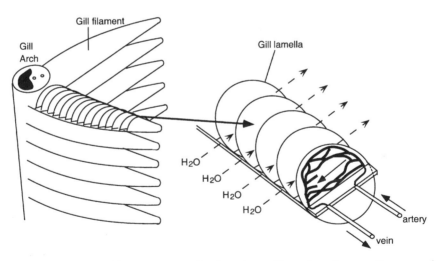

Figure 14.2. Gill lamella arrangement in the teleost. There is a large surface area for exchange, with many gill filaments each containing many gill lamellae. Note that the water and blood flow in opposite directions. (Adapted from Randall DJ. Control and coordination of gas exchange in water breathers. In: Boutilier RG, editor. *Advances in Comparative and Environmental Physiology*, vol 6, *Vertebrate Gas Exchange, From Environment to Cell*. New York: Springer-Verlag, 1990, p 264.)

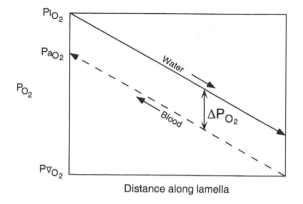

Figure 14.3. Countercurrent gas exchange in the fish gill. As water enters the gill, it releases O_2 via diffusion to the blood. Blood moving in the opposite direction picks up O_2 reaching a relatively high P_{O_2} before leaving the gill lamella. The P_{O_2} difference between water and blood is constant along the gill. (Adapted from Schmidt-Nielsen K. *Animal Physiology: Adaptation and Environment.* New York: Cambridge University Press, 1980, 1980, p. 21.)

density of water (compared with air) limits ventilation; the solubility of O_2 is much lower in water so a given tidal volume of water contains much less O_2; the diffusivity of O_2 and CO_2 is markedly reduced in water.

Reptilian Lungs

The lungs of reptiles are rudimentary in structure yet somewhat efficient in gas exchange. The lower energy demands of ectotherms (cold-blooded animals) allows these lower efficiency, gas exchange organs to fulfill their requirements. Reptilian lungs are either single chambered (unicameral), few chambered (paucicameral), or many chambered (multicameral), and they contrast with the alveolar mammalian lungs in that reptile lungs have a lower surface area for diffusional exchange.

The unicameral lungs of the Tegu lizard are essentially a pair of air bags. The walls are composed of a honeycomb-like arrangement of air tubes (faveoli) surrounded by walls of capillaries (Fig. 14.4). O_2 moves from a large air space in the middle of the lung into the tubes, presumably by diffusion. Although there are muscle bands around the lungs that may play a role in mixing, diffusion probably plays a greater role in the Tegu lung than in the mammalian lung. It is interesting that the diffusing capacity for O_2 (DL_{O_2}) of the Tegu lung is about 14% of the DL_{O_2} for human lungs (normalized for lung volume). The lower DL_{O_2} results from the relatively small capillary surface area. Yet the blood oxygenates well, perhaps because of an increased capillary transit time. In addition, the distribution of $\dot{V}_A/\dot{Q}$ is much more heterogeneous than that of mammalian lungs. Even though the

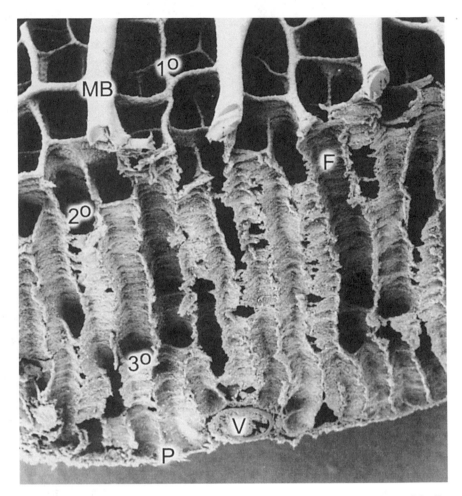

Figure 14.4. A scanning electron micrograph of the wall of the unicameral lung of the Tegu lizard. The pleura (P) is oriented at the bottom of the micrograph while at the top is a view looking obliquely down into the openings of the primary (1°) faveoli (F). Also shown are the secondary (2°) and tertiary (3°) faveoli. Muscle bands (MB) are arranged along this internal surface. A blood vessel (V) is seen just inside the outer surface of the lung. (From Hlastala MP et al. The matching of ventilation and perfusion in the lung of the Tegu lizard, *Tupinambis nigropunctatus. Respir Physiol* 60:277–294, 1985, with permission.)

unicameral lung is less efficient than the mammalian lung, gas exchange is sufficient because of the low O_2 demand of the animal.

Birds

Bird lungs contrast sharply with reptile lungs. Flying birds often have very high O_2 demands and must possess a very efficient gas exchange system, even in the face of the severe hypoxia that is encountered at altitude. Bird lungs use a highly efficient cross-current arrangement of noncompliant gas tubes (parabronchi) and blood vessels (Fig. 14.5). The flow of inspired gas is not fully understood, but is thought to be unidirectional through the parabronchi. During inspiration, air passes through the trachea and into the highly compliant caudal air sacs. Some of this initial inspiration passes through the neopulmonic parabronchi, resulting in some gas exchange. In addition, the air in the neopulmonic parabronchi moves into the cranial air sacs. During expiration, air from the caudal air sacs moves through the neopulmonic parabronchi into the paleopulmonic parabronchi. The air passes unidirectionally during both inspiration and expiration. In addition, air in the cranial air sacs is exhaled out the trachea. It is thought that an aerodynamic valving system

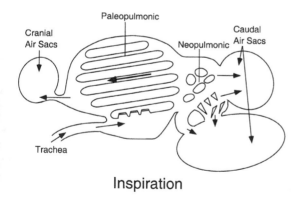

Inspiration

Figure 14.5. Schematic of the bird lung. During inspiration air passes through the trachea to the caudal air sacs and the neopulmonic lung. Air then passes through the parabronchi in the paleopulmonic lung, where gas exchange occurs, and into the cranial air sacs. Air is then exhaled through the trachea. The passage of air through the bird lung requires two respiratory cycles. (Adapted from Piiper J, Scheid P. Comparative physiology of respiration: Functional analysis of gas exchange organs in vertebrates. In: Widdecombe JG, editor. *International Review of Physiology: Respiratory Physiology II*, vol 14. Boston: University Park Press, 1977, pp. 220–253.)

at the base of the trachea causes the unidirectional flow of the bird lung. The cross-current arrangement of bird lungs allows the mixed end-pulmonary capillary blood to have a P_{O_2} exceeding the exhaled air P_{O_2}. This is a distinct advantage over mammals when exercising at high altitude with critically low inspired P_{O_2} values. The unique cross-current arrangement provides a means for increasing arterial P_{O_2} above exhaled air P_{O_2}, enhancing performance at high altitude.

Insects

Insects have a rigid exoskeleton making it impossible to ventilate lungs. Insects bring the external air into their bodies through a system with tube-like airways (Fig. 14.6). This network of tracheae makes contact with the outside environment through openings called *spiracles*. The network passes through the body and brings air within a short diffusion distance of all cells for the exchange of O_2 and CO_2. The smaller branches (tracheoles) are less than 1 μm in diameter, a size that allows air movement but would be too small for blood and red cells. Although a circulatory system is not needed for gas exchange, it can help with the transport of metabolic nutrients to the cells.

The spiracles have a closing mechanism that permits control of the exchange of O_2, CO_2, and water vapor. If an insect is exposed to high CO_2 or low O_2 levels,

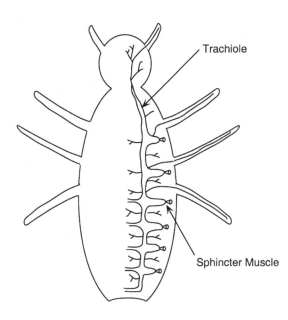

Trachiole

Sphincter Muscle

Figure 14.6. The trachiolar system of the insect carries O_2 to the tissues by diffusion through a series of tubes distributed through the body. There is some assistance from convection as sphincter muscles at the mouth of each trachiole facilitates gas movement as body movements compress and expand the trachioles. (Adapted from Wigglesworth VB. *The Principles of Insect Physiology*. London: Cambridge University Press, 1972, p. 358.)

the spiracles stay open, enhancing the exchange of O_2 and CO_2. This also, however, increases water exchange and will lead to dehydration within a short time.

The tracheae are relatively rigid and do not collapse. They are arranged in a folded manner so that changes in pressure can cause changes in tracheal volume and, in conjunction with the spiracles, create active ventilation. In some insects, ventilation is carried out by abdominal movements. During flight, pressure changes may be sufficient to expel up to two-thirds of the tracheolar volume in one exhalation.

Many aquatic insects take advantage of diffusional gas exchange in a unique way by taking along a store of air when they dive. The spiracular openings are hydrophobic and surrounded by hydrophobic hairs that help break the water surface to reestablish contact with the air on surfacing from a dive. Air carried along on the dive is held in place by nonwettable surfaces and hydrophobic hairs. Gas exchange is then carried out between the gas pocket and the water via diffusion. In some insects, a region of the body is covered with a dense array of relatively rigid hairs, creating a plastron (diffusional gill) that allows continual gas exchange. Although the gas pocket affords the opportunity to dive, it carries several liabilities. The bouyancy of the bubble requires the insect to use much more energy to dive. The depth of a dive affects the maximum duration because of the compression of the air pocket. Such diving can only occur in well-oxygenated water.

Skin-Gas Exchange

Amphibians use the skin for exchanging O_2 and CO_2. Many amphibians and a few salamanders rely solely on the skin for all their gas exchange requirements. In the amphibian skin, blood capillaries equilibrate with external air or water through a tissue diffusion barrier. In contrast to mammalian lungs, amphibian skin relies on diffusion as a primary component of the exchange process. Capillaries form a mesh-like network beneath the surface of the skin (Fig. 14.7). The diffusion barrier varies from species to species, but may be on the order of 25 to 100 μm thick.

The gas exchange across the skin can be locally regulated by altering the local blood flow. In frog skin, hypoxia reduces local blood flow, and hence gas exchange. This provides a compensatory mechanism that helps the frog optimize gas exchange in its local environment. Imagine a frog sitting in the mud with half of its body exposed to water or air. Because the mud presents such a large diffusion barrier, little O_2 would be available. Reduction in blood flow to that region of the skin in the mud allows the frog to direct more blood to the well-oxygenated skin in the air. This vasoconstriction mechanism is similar to hypoxic pulmonary vasoconstriction in the mammalian lung.

Because of a large body mass to skin surface area, all but the very smallest

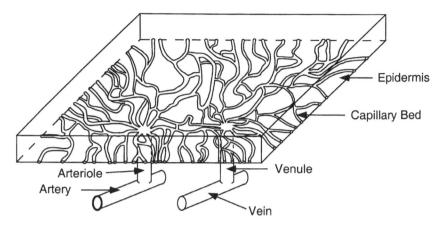

Figure 14.7. Schematic of the subsurface blood vessel arrangement in frog skin. The capillaries are arranged in a mesh-like pattern at a fixed distance from the surface. Diffusion is the only mechanism of exchange between the capillary bed and the surface. (Adapted from Malvin GM. Cardiovascular regulation of cutaneous gas exchange. In: Heatwole H, Barthalmus GT, editors. *Amphibian Biology,* vol 2, *The Integument.* Chipping Norton, Australia: Surrey Beatty & Sons, 1994, pp. 147–167, 1994.)

mammals are unable to take care of their gas exchange through the skin. It has recently been discovered, however, that a small newborn marsupial, the Julia Creek dunnart, about 4 mm in length and 17 mg in weight with a very thin, transparent skin, can take care of its entire metabolic O_2 demand by diffusion through the skin.

Oxygen-Carrying Proteins

Many invertebrates are able to carry sufficient O_2 in simple physical solution. These are animals that have very low O_2 requirements and live in cold environments (with increased physical solubility of O_2 and CO_2). Many animal species need to increase the O_2-carrying capacity of blood or hemolymph with respiratory pigments. In some cases, the pigment is dissolved in the blood fluid. In others, however, it is enclosed in cells, with none in the blood fluid. This serves the useful purpose of preventing loss of hemoglobin in the kidneys. The various types of respiratory pigment are listed in Table 14.1.

The relative O_2 affinity of hemoglobin varies in different animals living in different environmental conditions. Humans have a P_{50} of 27 mm Hg, for example, allowing suitable uptake of O_2 in the lungs at sea level and up to moderate altitudes and allowing adequate O_2 delivery to the tissues. Some animals that live at high

Table 14.1. Oxygen Carrying Pigments

PIGMENT	DESCRIPTION	MOLECULAR WEIGHT	ANIMAL SPECIES
Hemocyanin	Copper-based Carried in solution	300,000–9,000,000	Most molluscs; some arthropods (crabs, lobsters)
Hemerythrin	Iron-based Carried in cells	108,000	A few marine worms; some priapuloids
Chlorocruorin	Iron-porphyrin Carried in solution	2,750,000	Four families of marine polychete worms
Hemoglobin	Iron-porphyrin Carried in solution or cells	17,000–3,000,000	Most phyla

From Pierson DJ. The evolution of breathing: 5. Oxygen-carrying pigments: Respiratory mass transit. *Respir Care* 27: 963–970, 1982, with permission.

altitude (such as the llama and vicuna) have hemoglobin with increased O_2 affinity (decreased P_{50}), allowing adequate O_2 uptake in the lungs at altitudes of 16,000 ft ($P_B \approx 415$ mm Hg; see Fig. 11.1) while providing for tissue O_2 delivery. These animals have a greater capillary density (smaller diffusion distances) than humans, permitting O_2 diffusion to mitochondria at lower capillary P_{O_2} values.

Fetal blood has a lower P_{50} than maternal blood (see Chapter 12). This affords the advantage of allowing for a higher umbilical vein O_2 content even though the P_{O_2} is lower than maternal uterine venous P_{O_2}. This relationship is mandatory because there must be a P_{O_2} difference if O_2 is to diffuse from the maternal blood to the fetal blood.

Control of Respiration in Air Breathers

The production, integration, and optimization of respiratory movements in air breathers results from the central processing of inputs from different receptor groups. Some animals (mammals, birds, and fish) breathe in a continuous pattern while others (reptiles and amphibia) breathe in a periodic fashion.

There are insufficient data to distinguish among three possible mechanisms for central rhythm generation. The first is that all vertebrates possess a central rhythm generator (made up of either pacemaker cells or a central neuronal network) that operates at subthreshold levels requiring peripheral or higher central input to bring it to threshold. The second mechanism is that all aspects of respiratory pattern result from the integration of peripheral inputs. The third is that the control mechanisms are not common to all vertebrates and that central rhythm generators are present in animals that exhibit continuous breathing patterns but not in those that breathe in a periodic fashion. Although there is no uniform agreement on which of these mechanisms holds true, most scientists favor the first.

All air breathers exhibit a hypoxic ventilatory response, which is relatively flat over the normal physiological range and increases ventilation during hypoxia. Burrowing birds and mammals have a relatively blunted response, while highly aerobic mammals have a strong response.

The tissue associated with O_2 chemoreception is similar in all vertebrates. In mammals the carotid bodies are located at the bifurcations of the common carotid arteries into their internal and external branches. The aortic bodies are located in the region of the aortic arch and the roots of the major arteries of the thorax. In most lizards, the internal carotid artery arises from the common carotid arch by a variable number of openings forming communicating channels. In birds and turtles, chemoreceptive tissue is not present at the carotid bifurcation but rather in the central cardiovascular area close to the parathyroid and thyroid glands. In turtles the major aggregation of chemoreceptive tissue is located on the aortic arch.

The pattern of breathing varies among the species. Almost all reptiles exhibit periodic breathing. One pattern demonstrates ventilation in episodes separated by relatively long periods of breath-holding. In a second pattern, single breaths are separated by shorter intervals. In birds and reptiles, expiration is an active process. Mammals use passive expiration at rest and add expiratory muscle effort with exercise. In mammals, during periods of reduced metabolism such as sleep or hibernation, end-expiratory pauses (apneas) begin to appear. During hibernation, these periods can become prolonged, with pauses after expiration.

The hypercapnic ventilatory response varies considerably in magnitude over the different vertebrate species. Again, the burrowing species tend to have reduced hypercapnic ventilatory response. In birds and some reptiles, the hypercapnic ventilatory response may result from the response of intrapulmonary chemoreceptors within the lungs. The true nature of these intrapulmonary chemoreceptors has not yet, however, been fully characterized. Central chemoreceptors have been described in great detail in mammals near the ventrolateral surface of the medulla between the VIIth and XIIth cranial nerves. These central chemoreceptors respond to changes in the local hydrogen ion and CO_2 of the cerebral interstitial fluid (see Chapter 9). Studies are now revealing a similar process in birds and reptiles (see Milsom, 1990).

Scaling of Respiration Across the Animal Kingdom

The exchange of respiratory gases (O_2 and CO_2) depends to a great degree on the body size of the animal. Certainly larger animals must produce a greater amount of energy and thus have a greater $\dot{V}_{O_2}$ at rest. For birds and mammals, it has been determined that the relationship is exponentially related by the power of ¾:

$$\dot{V}_{O_2} = A \times BM^{\frac{3}{4}}$$

where A is a proportionality constant and BM is body mass. This relationship has generally been found to apply over the range of unicellular organisms to whales (18 orders of magnitude), including both ectotherm (cold-blooded) and endotherm (warm-blooded) species. Because less metabolic energy goes into maintaining body heat, ectotherms generally have a basal metabolic rate (BMR) of between 2.5% and 5% of the endotherm species of similar body weight. In addition, the BMR varies from the standard line depending on individual environmental or behavioral needs. Marsupials are about 30% lower in BMR than are similar-sized mammals. Seals and whales have a BMR about twice expected because of the need to maintain body temperature in cold waters.

Many respiratory parameters adhere to a similar relationship with body weight (Fig. 14.8). These include tidal volume and expiratory ventilation. Not surprisingly, there is also a similar relationship with ventilatory frequency. The exponent for this ventilation frequency, however, is -0.25. Further details about this respiratory scaling over the animal kingdom can be found in Dejours, (1975).

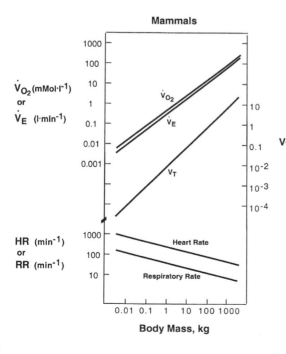

Figure 14.8. Relationship between physiological variables and body mass. Oxygen consumption, $\dot{V}_{O_2}$; ventilation, $\dot{V}_E$; tidal volume, V_T; heart (HR) and respiratory (RR) rates as functions of body mass of mammals ranging in size from 4 gm to 4 tons. (Adapted from Dejours P. *Principles of Comparative Respiratory Physiology.* Amsterdam: North-Holland/American Elsevier, 1975.)

Further Reading

1. Cameron JN. *The Respiratory Physiology of Animals*. New York: Oxford University Press, 1989.
2. Dejours P. *Principles of Comparative Respiratory Physiology*. New York: American Elsevier, 1975.
3. Schmidt-Nielsen K. *Animal Physiology: Adaptation and Environment*. 2nd ed. New York: Cambridge University Press, 1979.
4. Milsom WK. Control and co-ordination of gas exchange in air breathers. In: Boutilier RG, editor. *Advances in Comparative and Environmental Physiology*, vol 6. Berlin: Springer-Verlag, 1990.
5. Mortola JP et al. Breathing through the skin in a newborn mammal. *Nature* 397:660, 1999.

Study Questions

14.1. How does countercurrent blood and water flow help to improve gas exchange efficiency of gills?

14.2. Why is the reptile lung less efficient than the mammalian lung?

14.3. How does the bird lung allow the arterial P_{O_2} to be greater than mixed exhaled P_{O_2}?

14.4. How does a hemoglobin with increased O_2 affinity help survival at high altitude?

14.5. Describe the insect respiratory apparatus.

Answers to Study Questions

Chapter 1

1.1. In a gas mixture, the pressure exerted by each individual gas species is referred to as its *partial pressure.*

1.2. The vapor pressure of a gas over a liquid is the partial pressure exerted by gas molecules when there is an equilibrium between the liquid and gas phases for these molecules.

1.3. The amount of gas that can dissolve in a liquid is directly proportional to the partial pressure of that gas above the liquid.

1.4. A total of 0.282ml $O_2 \cdot dl^{-1}$ of plasma will be dissolved because the amount dissolved is the product of the solubility coefficient (0.00282 ml $O_2 \cdot dl^{-1} \cdot mm\ Hg^{-1}$) times the O_2 partial pressure of 100 mm Hg.

1.5. In a flow system addition of a parallel flow resistance will reduce the total resistance. The addition of a series flow resistance will increase the total resistance.

1.6. In laminar flow in a tube the resistance to flow is inversely proportional to the fourth power of the radius. The resistance will increase 16-fold if the radius is halved.

1.7. The subject's arterial O_2 concentration can be determined by solving equation 1.16 for Ca_{O_2}.

$$\dot{Q} = \frac{\dot{V}_{O_2}}{Ca_{O_2} - Cv_{O_2}} \tag{1.16}$$

$$Ca_{O_2} = \frac{\dot{V}_{O_2}}{\dot{Q}} + Cv_{O_2}$$

This results in a Ca_{O_2} of 190 ml $O_2 \cdot l\ blood^{-1}$.

1.8. Molecular diffusion is the transport of a species from a region of high concentration to one of low concentration.

1.9. Ṁ is directly proportional to the cross-sectional area and inversely related to the thickness of the membrane.

Chapter 2

2.1. By warming and humidifying inspired air.

2.2. Generations 0 through 11.

2.3. Generations 0 through 16.

2.4. Between generations 16 and 17.

2.5. The sheet flow concept visualized the capillary bed as a sheet of blood with posts of membrane, providing structure. The hydrodynamic resistance to blood flow is lower than it is in a parallel group of small tubes.

2.6. The tracheal and bronchoesophageal arteries originate from the aorta and feed the trachea, bronchi, and bronchioles. Blood from the trachea and large bronchi drain into the azygos vein. Smaller bronchi and bronchioles drain into the pulmonary circulation.

2.7. Inspiratory muscles serve to raise the ribs and expand the chest wall. The diaphragm contracts, dropping down to expand the lung volume. During normal quiet expiration, both inspiratory and expiratory muscles are relaxed. During forced exhalation, expiratory muscles pull the ribs down and inward while the abdominal muscles contract, raising the diaphragm.

Chapter 3

3.1. Reduced lung volume at any transpleural pressure with a normal chest wall curve will be the result in this restrictive disease. Reduced TLC, FRC, and RV will also occur.

3.2. Inspiratory effort capability is exceeded when water pressure exceeds 100 cm H_2O or 100 cm depth. A larger tube increases dead space. A smaller tube increases resistance.

3.3. With low surfactant, alveolar liquid surface tension increases, causing alveolar collapse as small alveoli empty into large alveoli.

3.4. Positive pleural pressure during forced exhalation causes airway collapse, increasing airway resistance.

3.5. In obstructive disease, R_{aw}, TLC, FRC, and RV are increased, while FEV_1/VC is reduced. In restrictive disease, TLC, FRC, and RV are decreased, while FEV_1/VC is normal or possibly increased.

3.6. Compliance (total thoracic)

$$= \frac{\Delta V}{\Delta P} = \frac{0.8 \text{ l}}{24 - 0 \text{ cm } H_2O} = 0.033 \text{ l} \cdot \text{cm } H_2O^{-1}$$

(Normal compliance would be about 0.1 l $\cdot$ cm H_2O^{-1}.) The peak pressure (30 cm H_2O) reflects elastic + flow resistive pressure (due to resistance in tubing, endotracheal tube tube, or airways.) Pleural pressure is determined as follows:

$$\text{Lung recoil} = \text{alveolar} - \text{pleural}$$
$$25 = 24 - (-1)$$

3.7. Alveolar pressure is obtained as follows:

$$\text{Lung recoil} = \text{alveolar} - \text{pleural (esophageal)}$$
$$5 = -2 - (-7)$$

(Normal is < 2.5 cm $H_2O \cdot l^{-1} \cdot$ sec.) If resistance does not change, an expiratory flow of 0.4 l $\cdot$ sec^{-1} will require an alveolar driving pressure of $0.4 \times 4 = 1.6$ cm H_2O. At the same lung volume, recoil pressure will be 5, so

$$\text{Lung recoil} = \text{alveolar} - \text{pleural}$$
$$5 = 1.6 - (-3.4)$$

Chapter 4

4.1. Inspired air picks up water and heat from the airway surface. The increased water vapor content reduces the inspired P_{O_2} and P_{N_2} until saturation is reached well into the airway tree. Increased air temperature has no effect on gas partial pressure except when increased air temperature allows greater uptake of water vapor.

4.2. With voluntary changes in ventilation, hypoventilation results in increased PA_{CO_2} and decreased PA_{CO_2}, while hyperventilation results in decreased PA_{CO_2} and increased PA_{CO_2}. Increases in ventilation during exercise are accompanied by comparable increases in metabolism, resulting in no change in alveolar gases.

4.3. Increases in R cause an increase in PA_{O_2}, whereas decreases in R cause a decrease in PA_{O_2}.

4.4. Alveolar P_{O_2} varies with an amplitude of about 4.5 mm Hg. Alveolar PA_{CO_2} has a smaller oscillation of about 2.5 mm Hg due to the buffering effect of lung tissues. Because the sum of gases must always equal atmospheric pressure, P_{N_2} also oscillates in response to the differences between $P_{A_{O_2}}$ and $P_{A_{CO_2}}$.

4.5. $\dfrac{V_D}{V_T} = \dfrac{Pa_{CO_2} - PE_{CO_2}}{Pa_{CO_2}} = \dfrac{40\text{mm Hg} - 25\text{mm Hg}}{40\text{mm Hg}} = 0.375$

V_D/V_T decreases with exercise.

4.6. Aerosols of 0.03, 0.3, 3, and 30 μm diameter would be found in alveoli, alveoli, nasal, and nasal regions, respectively.

4.7. A. Total ventilation $= 10 \times 750 = 7500$ ml · min^{-1} = 7.5 l · min^{-1}.
Alveolar ventilation $= 10 \times (750 - 300) = 4500$ ml · min^{-1} = 4.5 l · min^{-1}.
Wasted ventilation $= 10 \times 300 = 3000$ ml · min^{-1} = 3.0 l · min^{-1}

Alveoli expand by the full tidal volume (750 ml) not just by the alveolar or gas exchange portion of each breath. The anatomical and apparatus dead spaces are in series with the alveoli so that the alveoli first receive recycled gas from the prior exhalation (300 ml in this case) and then 450ml of fresh inspired gas capable of gas exchange with the blood.

B. $\dot{V}_E \cdot PE_{CO_2} = \dot{V}_A \cdot PA_{CO_2} + \dot{V}_D \cdot 0$

$PE_{CO_2} = \dfrac{4500}{7500} \cdot 40 = 24$ mm Hg

4.8. A. $\dfrac{V_D}{V_T} = \dfrac{Pa_{CO_2} - PE_{CO_2}}{Pa_{CO_2}} = \dfrac{50 - 30}{50} = 0.4$

$V_D = 0.4 \cdot V_T = 0.4 \cdot 500 = 200$ ml

B. $\dot{V}_A = \dot{V}_E - \dot{V}_D = f(V_T - V_D)$
$= 15(500 - 200) = 15 \times 300 = 4500$
$= 4.5$ l · min^{-1}

C. $\dot{V}_{CO_2} = \dot{V}_E \cdot FE_{CO_2}$ or $\dot{V}_A \cdot FA_{CO_2}$

$= f \cdot V_T \cdot \dfrac{PE_{CO_2}}{P_B - 47}$ or $\dot{V}_A \cdot \dfrac{PA_{CO_2}}{P_B - 47}$

$= 15 \cdot 500 \cdot \dfrac{30}{713}$ or $4.5 \cdot \dfrac{50}{713}$

$= 316$ ml · min^{-1} or 0.316 l · min^{-1}

Chapter 5

5.1.

$$P_{avg} = P_{diastolic} + \frac{1}{3}(P_{systolic} - P_{diastolic})$$

$$P_{pa} = 6 + \frac{1}{3}(25 - 6) \cong 12.3 \text{ mm Hg}$$

$$P_{sa} = 80 + \frac{1}{3}(120 - 80) \cong 93.3 \text{ mm Hg}$$

$$\frac{R_p}{R_s} = \frac{\dfrac{\Delta P_p}{\dot{Q}}}{\dfrac{\Delta P_s}{\dot{Q}}} = \frac{P_{pa} - P_{pv}}{P_{sa} - P_{sv}} = \frac{12 - 0}{93 - 5} = \frac{12}{88} \cong 0.14$$

5.2. It has been thought that gravity influences the distribution of pulmonary blood flow via an influence on pulmonary vascular pressures. The four-zone model assumes that vascular pressures increase lower in the lung because of the weight of blood above. It also assumes that the vascular pressure decreases higher in the lung, changing in proportion to height up the lung as determined by the density of blood. In zone 1, alveolar pressure exceeds both arterial and venous pressure compressing the alveolar capillaries, resulting in zero blood flow. In zone 2, arterial pressure exceeds alveolar pressure, which exceeds venous pressure. Pulmonary blood flow increases with descent into zone 2. In zone 3, both arterial and venous pressures exceed alveolar pressure, causing all capillaries to be open. The result should be a decreasing flow with increasing height within the lungs. Measurements of blood flow to small regions of the lung demonstrate a decreasing flow with ascent up the lung but a great amount of heterogeneity within any isogravitational plane; thus the argument can be made that gravity has little influence on pulmonary blood flow distribution.

5.3. In the event of low ventilation to a region, alveolar hypoxia causes vasoconstriction to decrease flow and return blood gases in that region toward normal.

5.4. Interstitial and perivascular pressures, plasma and interstitial fluid osmotic pressures, vascular permeability, and filtration coefficient all play a role in the formation of pulmonary edema.

5.5. Positive end-expiratory pressure increases mean alveolar pressure, which in turn increases pulmonary capillary resistance and, hence, pulmonary vascular resistance and pulmonary artery pressure.

Chapter 6

6.1. Saturation is unchanged, and O_2 content is reduced by 20%

6.2. Decreased pH, increased CO_2, increased temperature or increased 2,3-diphosphoglycerate $\rightarrow$ increased P_{50}.

6.3. CO_2 is stored in the blood through physical solution in plasma and the HCO_3^- created by hydration within the red cell and carbamino bound to hemoglobin.

6.4. The Bohr effect accounts for 2% of O_2 exchange, whereas the Haldane effect accounts for 40% of CO_2 exchange.

6.5. Measure $\dot{V}_{O_2}$ and sample arterial and mixed venous (pulmonary arterial) O_2 content.

6.6. Aerobic metabolism.

6.7. In the tissue, uptake of CO_2 causes a rightward shift in the O_2 equilibrium curve, allowing a greater release of O_2 (lower venous O_2 content) at the same venous P_{O_2} (diffusion driving pressure). Similarly, release of O_2 shifts the CO_2 equilibrium curve to the left, allowing greater CO_2 uptake at the same P_{CO_2}. The opposite occurs in the lungs.

6.8. An increase in tissue perfusion would lead to an increase in tissue P_{O_2}. A decrease in hematocrit will decrease tissue P_{O_2}.

6.9. Exercise creates an increase in O_2 demand that can be compensated for via increased tissue perfusion, an enhanced role of the Bohr effect due to increased CO_2 production, and/or recruitment of additional capillaries to reduce diffusion distances.

Chapter 7

7.1. The β_m/β_b ratio.

7.2. CO has a very low β_m/β_b ratio.

7.3. $Pa_{O_2} > 150$ mm Hg, 100% O_2 breathing, and normal cardiac output.

7.4. The sum of partial pressures of gases in the gas phase is greater than the sum of partial pressure in venous blood or the tissue phase.

7.5. The nonlinearity of the O_2 equilibrium curve amplifies $(A - a)P_{O_2}$.

7.6. Increasing heterogeneity worsens any gas exchange process.

7.7. A. $PI_{O_2} = 150$ mm Hg $\rightarrow$ no effect of altitude or low FI_{O_2}.

   B. $P_{CO_2} = 50$ mm Hg $\rightarrow$ some hypoventilation, but if ventilation were corrected to $P_{CO_2} = 40$ mm Hg, then P_{O_2} would increase to about 60 mm Hg (which is still hypoxemic).

   C. $DL_{CO} = 90$% predicted $\rightarrow$ within normal range, no diffusion limitation.

D. Breathing 100% O_2, $(A - a)P_{O_2} \cong 300$ mm Hg $\rightarrow$ 15% shunt.

E. The 15% shunt and the mild hypoventilation would not explain the large $(A - a)\ P_{O_2}$ of 50 mm Hg breathing air. Thus there is probably some $\dot{V}_A/\dot{Q}$ abnormality present as well.

Chapter 8

8.1. Respiratory rate decreases, and inspiratory time increases. There is a deepening of inspiration—that is, tidal volume increases.

8.2. In apneusis inspiratory time is markedly prolonged. Apneusis results from a lesion of the pontine respiratory group and cutting of the vagus nerves.

8.3. Dorsal respiratory group and ventral respiratory group.

8.4. P-cells act as sensory relay neurons of slowly adapting pulmonary stretch receptors; they are not driven by central inspiratory activity.

8.5. Nucleus parabrachialis medialis and the Kölliker-Fusé nucleus.

8.6. C3 to C5.

8.7. Ventrolateral columns.

8.8. Network and pacemaker models.

Chapter 9

9.1. Type I or glomus cell.

9.2. A Pa_{O_2} decrease, a Pa_{CO_2} increase, and a pH decrease.

9.3. Ventilation and PA_{O_2} are related to each other by a nonlinear relationship. It is best described by a hyperbolic function; specifically, ventilation is inversely related to PA_{O_2}:

$$\dot{V} = V_0 + \frac{A}{(PA_{O_2} - 32)}$$

9.4. Breathing would increase due to activation of central chemosensors.

9.5. The blood–brain barrier has a low permeability to ions, but CO_2 is freely diffusible through it. Thus rapid elevation of Pa_{CO_2} can readily stimulate breathing via central chemosensor activation; in contrast, rapid elevation in arterial hydrogen ion is not an effective stimulus to the central chemosensors.

9.6. Pa_{CO_2}.

9.7. Peripheral chemosensors are stimulated, and central chemosensors are depressed.

Chapter 10

10.1. The diving reflex, which can be initiated by water instilled in the nose or applied to the face, includes a number of responses: apnea, laryngeal closure, bronchoconstriction, bradycardia, and vasoconstriction of some vascular beds such as skin, muscle, and kidney.

10.2. Slowly adapting receptors; rapidly adapting receptors; pulmonary C-fiber endings; bronchial C-fiber endings.

10.3. Activation of slowly adapting receptors is responsible for the Hering-Breuer inflation reflex. Maintained lung inflation during expiration causes a marked increase in expiratory phase duration. Also overall increases in lung volume will act to inhibit breathing, that is, respiratory rate will decrease.

10.4. Activation of these rapidly adapting receptors will produce cough, mucus, and bronchoconstriction.

10.5. Activation of C-fiber endings is responsible for the pulmonary chemo-reflex inflation reflex. This reflex involves bradycardia, hypotension, and apnea.

10.6. Parasympathetic activity increases airway smooth muscle tone.

10.7. The i-NANC system is made up of peptide-containing nerve fibers that appear to arise from parasympathetic ganglia. One of the peptides that is associated with the i-NANC system is vasoactive intestinal peptide (VIP). VIP has been shown to relax airway smooth muscle.

Chapter 11

11.1. Approximately 5000 m.

11.2. Ventilatory acclimatization is the time-dependent increase in ventilation that occurs in response to continuing hypoxemia resulting from exposure to altitude.

11.3. Ventilation will diminish abruptly, but it will remain elevated compared with its normal value at sea level.

11.4. Blood adaptations include increased hematocrit and hemoglobin concentration and elevated levels of 2,3-diphosphoglycerate.

11.5. This increase in the alveolar–arterial difference under conditions of exercise at high altitude appears to be due mostly to a diffusion limitation.

11.6. The volume is taken from 2 to 3 ATA. The new volume, then, will be 0.67 l.

11.7. The body has a number of compartments with different washin/washout time constants. The fast compartments absorb gas more rapidly and are more likely to be supersaturated early in the washout. The slow compartments are more likely to be supersaturated late in washout.

11.8. The sum of partial pressures in the gas phase is greater than the sum of partial pressures in the blood or tissue phase.

11.9. Theory indicates that lipid membranes are compressed by absolute pressure and expanded by dissolved inert gases.

11.10. Increased P_{O_2} helps to drive CO off of hemoglobin and increases O_2 content in physical solution. High inspired P_{O_2} leads to pulmonary O_2 toxicity.

Chapter 12

12.1. Maximal O_2 consumption during exercise can be limited by cardiac output, arterial O_2 content, which is governed by the respiratory system, and venous O_2 content, which is governed by O_2 extraction by the exercising muscle.

12.2. Arterial P_{O_2}, P_{CO_2}, and pH do not change during mild to moderate exercise from their levels during resting control conditions.

12.3. During heavy exercise increased levels of plasma [H^+], norepinephrine, and K^+ may contribute to the increased respiratory drive.

12.4. This disequilibrium results from the enhanced capability through training of the cardiovascular system to increase cardiac output and therefore pulmonary blood flow to very high levels. Arterial hypoxemia is explained by the presence of disequilibrium between alveolar and end-pulmonary capillary P_{O_2}. The mechanism possibly involves insufficient time to achieve equilibrium between alveolar gas and capillary blood, as the transit time of red blood cells within the pulmonary capillaries is decreased.

12.5. The two main sleep states are called nonrapid eye movement (NREM), or quiet, sleep and rapid eye movement (REM) sleep, sometimes called active or desynchronized sleep. NREM is characterized by varying degrees of large-amplitude electroencephalographic activity and the presence of tonic electromyographic activity. REM is characterized by bursts of rapid eye movements, a desynchronized electroencephalographic activity, dreaming, and a loss of muscle tone.

12.6. During both NREM and REM sleep, overall ventilation decreases compared with the awake state.

12.7. Obstructive sleep apnea is the cessation of airflow for a period of time at the mouth and nostrils. This involves a closure of the upper airway at the level of the oropharynx despite the presence of respiratory efforts by the main muscles of breathing. Airway closure can depend on anatomical factors such as variations in size of the upper airway opening, as well as the balance of forces on the upper airways as gas goes in and out of the airway (Bernoulli effect). Also, sleep state can profoundly influence airway closure. In REM sleep there is a marked loss of tonic and inspiratory phase–linked activity in the genioglossus muscle. This loss in activity coincides with a profound reduction in tidal volume, which points to the possible role of sleep state and loss of tone in the tongue muscle as potential causes of some forms of obstructive sleep apnea.

12.8. The three key structures of the fetal circulatory system that channel oxygenated blood from the placenta into the aorta for distribution to the vital organs are the ductus arteriosus, the foramen ovale, and the ductus venosus.

12.9. HbA is composed of α- and β-chains. In contrast, in HbF, ρ-chains replace β-chains. Functionally, HbF has a much greater affinity for O_2 than does HbA.

12.10. Immature lungs show a pressure–volume curve where the initial inflation curve is similar to that seen in mature lungs, but the lungs collapse at zero pressure on deflation. The inflation and deflation curves for the second breath are the same as for the first. Large opening pressures are required, and at the end of deflation the lungs collapse. In mature lungs the first inflation requires a large trans-lung pressure to instill a significant amount of air into the lungs (called the *opening pressure*); with additional pressure, the lungs easily fill to capacity. The deflation curve is separated from the inflation curve, thus exhibiting hysteresis. At zero pressure the lungs retain about 25% of their total volume. The second inflation shows that no opening pressure is required to initiate inflation of the lungs, and at the opening pressure of the first breath the lungs are now filled with about 80% of total volume.

Chapter 13

13.1. A buffer value is the negative of the reciprocal of the slope of the titration curve at any given pH.

13.2. The following four systems are among the important buffer systems in the body: H_2CO_3/HCO_3^- and $H_2PO_4^-/HPO_4^=$ in the plasma and extracellular fluid; HHb/Hb^- in red blood cells; and $HCO_3^-/CO_3^=$ in bone.

13.3. Hemoglobin is an effective buffer because (*1*) it is in high concentration in red blood cells; (*2*) because imidazole groups are present on the hemoglobin molecule, the pK of hemoglobin (6.8) is close to the normal blood pH range; and (*3*) hemoglobin O_2 saturation alters the buffering capacity of hemoglobin. In this case, when P_{O_2} is low, as in the systemic capillaries, the H^+ affinity is high; the converse occurs in the pulmonary capillary where the P_{O_2} is high.

13.4. When P_{CO_2} is changed, there will be a larger change in pH occurring for blood *in vivo* than for blood *in vitro* because of several factors: (*1*) blood contains a number of effective buffers including plasma proteins and hemoglobin; (*2*) the interstitial compartment contains essentially no protein buffers and thus behaves like a pure bicarbonate solution; (*3*) bicarbonate and CO_2 are in equilibrium between the blood and the interstitial compartment; and (*4*) in the total extracellular fluid volume (including blood) the blood is only about one-third of the volume, the remainder being the interstitial volume.

13.5. In response to chronic respiratory acidosis there will be a metabolic alkalosis compensation, and plasma bicarbonate will rise.

13.6. In response to chronic metabolic acidosis, ventilatory compensation is not of itself capable of fully returning the pH of blood to 7.4 because the compensation mechanism involves an increase in ventilation with an offsetting reduction in arterial P_{CO_2}. The latter acts as a brake on ventilation.

13.7. To determine the base excess, you can use a Davenport diagram or the following steps:

    1. Solve the Henderson-Hasselbalch relationship (Eq. 13.9) for pH given a P_{CO_2} of 30 mm Hg and a $[HCO_3^-]$ of 15 mEq $\cdot$ l^{-1}. This results is a pH of 7.32.

    2. With a buffer value of 10 sl, the change in $[HCO_3^-]$ to make the pH equal to 7.4 is

$$\Delta[HCO_3^-] = -10 \times \Delta pH = -10(7.4 - 7.32) = -0.8 \text{ mEq} \cdot l^{-1}$$

$$[HCO_3^-] = 15 - 0.8 = 14.2 \text{ mEq} \cdot l^{-1}$$

    3. The base excess is $14.2 - 24 \cong -10$ mEq $\cdot$ l^{-1}; therefore, because the base excess is less than -3 mEq $\cdot$ l^{-1}, there is a component of metabolic acidosis.

Chapter 14

14.1. With a countercurrent flow of blood and water, blood leaving the capillary exchanges with entering water, which has the highest P_{O_2}.

14.2. The reptile lung has very little convective gas mixing. Diffusion becomes the limiting process.

14.3. In the cross-current system, blood is equilibrated, with gas having a

P_{O_2} anywhere between parabronchus P_{O_2} and end-air capillary P_{O_2}. The mixed blood P_{O_2} exceeds exhaled P_{O_2}.

14.4. It allows greater arterial O_2 content even with lower alveolar P_{O_2} of high altitude.

14.5. The insect has a network of spiracles and tracheoles that takes outside air through the body by diffusion.

Appendix A

Symbols Used in Respiratory Physiology

atm	Atmosphere
f	Frequency
ℓ	Length (m, cm, mm, μm)
l	Liter
n	Number of moles of gas
r	Radius
sl	slyke
v	Velocity
A	Area
BE	Base excess
C	Content or concentration of a substance in the blood (ml · dl^{-1})
C_{cw}	Compliance of the chest wall (l · cm H_2O^{-1})
C_L	Compliance of the lung (l · cm H_2O^{-1})
C_T	Compliance of the lung and chest wall together (l · cm H_2O^{-1})
C_{sp}	Specific compliance (l · cm H_2O^{-1} · l^{-1})
CA	Carbonic anhydrase
CO_2	Carbon dioxide
CO	Carbon monoxide
COHb	Carboxyhemoglobin
$\mathcal{D}$	Molecular diffusion coefficient
D	Diffusing capacity (ml · min^{-1} · mm Hg^{-1})
E	Expiratory
ERV	Expiratory reserve volume
F_X	Fractional concentration of a gas specie X
FRC	Functional residual capacity

H^+	Hydrogen ion
Hb	Hemoglobin
H_2O	Water
HCO_3^-	Bicarbonate ion
I	Inspiratory
IC	Inspiratory capacity
IRV	Inspiratory reserve volume
J	Flux
K_f	Filtration coefficient
L	Lung
M	Mass
$\dot{M}$	Mass flow rate
N_2	Nitrogen
N_{Re}	Reynolds number
NH_3	Ammonia
O_2	Oxygen
O_2Hb	Oxyhemoglobin
P	Pressure of a gas (mm Hg, cm H_2O, kPa)
$\mathscr{P}_X$	Membrane permeability of species X
P_X	Partial pressure of species X (mm Hg)
PVR	Pulmonary vascular resistance (mm Hg $\cdot$ l^{-1} $\cdot$ min)
R	Gas constant (0.08205 l $\cdot$ atm $\cdot$ mole^{-1} $\cdot$ °K^{-1} or 62.32 l $\cdot$ mm Hg $\cdot$ mole^{-1} $\cdot$ °K^{-1})
R	Gas exchange ratio
R	Resistance
RAR	Rapidly adapting receptor
RQ	Respiratory quotient
RV	Residual volume
S	Saturation in the blood (%)
SAR	Slowly adapting receptor
Q	Volume of blood (ml, l)
$\dot{Q}$	Blood flow (ml $\cdot$ min^{-1}, l $\cdot$ s^{-1})
T	Temperature (°C, °F, °K)
TLC	Total lung capacity (ml, l)
V	Volume of a gas (ml, l)
$\dot{V}$	Flow of gas (ml $\cdot$ min^{-1}, l $\cdot$ s^{-1})
$\dot{V}_{CO2}$	Metabolic production rate of CO_2 (ml CO_2 $\cdot$ min^{-1})
$\dot{V}_{O2}$	Metabolic consumption rate of O_2 (ml O_2 $\cdot$ min^{-1})
VC	Vital capacity
W	Work
β	Solubility coefficient (ml $\cdot$ dl^{-1} $\cdot$ mm Hg^{-1})

γ	Surface tension
η	Viscosity
Θ	A chemical reaction term
λ_x	Partition coefficient of species X
π_p	Plasma osmotic pressure
ρ	Density
σ	Osmotic reflection coefficient

Modifiers to Symbols

a	Arterial
A	Alveolar
atm	Atmospheric
B	Barometric
b	Blood
c	End capillary
D	Dead space
E	Expired
$\bar{E}$	Mixed expired
g	Gas
G	Inert gas
I	Inspired
la	Left atrial
M	Membrane
P	Plasma
pa	Pulmonary arterial
pl	Pleural
s	Shunt
t	Total
tis	Tissue
T	Tidal
v	Venous
$\bar{v}$	Mixed venous
X	Any particular gas species

Appendix B

Respiratory Parameters—Normal Values

Pulmonary Mechanics

P_{pl}	Pleural pressure	at FRC	-5	cm H_2O
		at TLC	-30	cm H_2O
C_T	Compliance of thorax		0.1	$1 \cdot$ cm H_2O^{-1}
C_{CW}	Compliance of chest wall		0.2	$1 \cdot$ cm H_2O^{-1}
C_L	Compliance of lungs		0.2	$1 \cdot$ cm H_2O^{-1}
R_{aw}	Airway resistance		<2.5	cm $H_2O \cdot 1^{-1} \cdot$ sec

Ventilation and Gas Transport

f	Respiratory frequency	12–15	per min
$\dot{V}_A$	Alveolar ventilation	4–5	$1 \cdot$ min^{-1}
$\dot{V}_E$	Total ventilation	6–8	$1 \cdot$ min^{-1}
V_T	Tidal volume	500	ml
V_{Danat}	Anatomical dead space volume	150–200	ml
V_D/V_T	Physiological dead space to tidal volume ratio	<0.4	
$\dot{V}_{O_2}$	Oxygen consumption	250–300	ml $\cdot$ min^{-1}
$\dot{V}_{CO_2}$	Carbon dioxide production	200–250	ml $\cdot$ min^{-1}
R	Respiratory exchange ratio	0.8	
$\dot{Q}$ or $\dot{Q}_T$	Cardiac output (total)	5	$1 \cdot$ min^{-1}
$\dot{Q}_S/\dot{Q}_T$	Shunt fraction	<5	%
Hb	Hemoglobin concentration	15	gm $\cdot$ dl^{-1}
P_{50}	Partial pressure of O_2 at 50% Hb sat	27	mm Hg

Blood Gas Values

PA_{O_2}	Alveolar partial pressure of O_2	100	mm Hg
PA_{CO_2}	Alveolar partial pressure of CO_2	40	mm Hg
Pa_{O_2}	Arterial partial pressure of O_2	90 ± 10	mm Hg
Pa_{CO_2}	Arterial partial pressure of CO_2	40 ± 3	mm Hg
Ca_{O_2}	Arterial content of O_2	20	$ml \cdot dl^{-1}$
$C\bar{v}_{O_2}$	Mixed venous content of O_2	15	$ml \cdot dl^{-1}$
$C(a-\bar{v})_{O_2}$	Arterial–venous O_2 content difference	5	$ml \cdot dl^{-1}$
Ca_{CO_2}	Arterial content of CO_2	47	$ml \cdot dl^{-1}$
$C\bar{v}_{CO_2}$	Mixed venous content of CO_2	51	$ml \cdot dl^{-1}$
$P\bar{v}_{O_2}$	Mixed venous partial pressure of O_2	40	mm Hg
$P\bar{v}_{CO_2}$	Mixed venous partial pressure of CO_2	46	mm Hg
pHa	Arterial pH	7.40 ± 0.03	Units
HCO_3^-	Arterial blood bicarbonate concentration	24 ± 2	$mEq \cdot l^{-1}$
BE	Base excess	0 ± 3	$mEq \cdot l^{-1}$

Pulmonary Function Tests

		25-year-old, 6 ft tall male	55-year-old, 5 ft tall female	Units
VC	Vital capacity	5.4	2.4	l
FRC	Functional residual capacity	4.0	2.2	l
RV	Residual volume	1.9	1.4	l
TLC	Total lung capacity	7.3	3.8	l
FEV_1	Forced expired volume in 1.0 second	4.4	2.0	l
FEV_1/VC	FEV_1/vital capacity ratio	80	75	%
DL_{CO}	Diffusing capacity for CO	36.0	18.0	$ml \cdot min^{-1}$ $mm\ Hg^{-1}$

Index